John Tanner is a practitioner in orthopaedic medicine and runs a sports injuries clinic. After qualifying in medicine and psychology in London he trained as a family practitioner, but enthusiasm for active and preventive therapy led him to follow post-graduate training in medical and osteopathic methods of manipulation, physical fitness training and the rehabilitation of the injured sportsman. As medical adviser to Champneys health resort in Hertfordshire on both clinical and policy issues, joining the BHMA at its inaugural conference was a natural progression. He is on the councils of both the Society and the Institute of Orthopaedic Medicine and actively supports the work of the Back Pain Association.

THE BRITISH HOLISTIC MEDICAL ASSOCIATION

BEATING BACK PAIN

Dr John Tanner
MB BS BSc

SERIES EDITOR

Dr Patrick C. Pietroni
MB BS FRCGP MRCP

DORLING KINDERSLEY · LONDON

Senior editor Jemima Dunne

Art editor Philip Lord

Editor Claire Le Bas

Designer Joanna Martin

Managing editor Daphne Razazan

First published in Great Britain in 1987 by
Dorling Kindersley Publishers Limited
9 Henrietta Street, London WC2E 8PS

Dedication by kind permission of
Northern Songs, copyright 1969.

reprinted 1992, 1994, 1996. (twice)

Visit us on the World Wide Web at
http://www.dk.com

British Library Cataloguing in Publication Data

Tanner, John
  Beating back pain.
  1. Backache
  I. Title
  616.7'306   RD768

ISBN 0-86318-224-0 Hardback
ISBN 0-86318-163-5 Paperback

Printed at Thomson Press (India) Ltd.

Contents

Introduction 7

1 ▤ Who gets back trouble? 10
WHO IS MOST AT RISK? 10
HIGH RISK OCCUPATIONS 13
PSYCHOLOGICAL FACTORS 14
YOUR OWN BACK PAIN 16

2 ▤ The healthy back 17
THE SPINE 17
THE SPINAL CANAL 21
LIGAMENTS AND MUSCLES 23
FUNCTIONS OF THE SPINE 27

3 ▤ Making your own diagnosis 28
LOWER BACK AND LEG PAIN 29
MID BACK PAIN 32
NECK, SHOULDER AND ARM PAIN 34

4 ▤ Acute and chronic back pain 36
DISC PROBLEMS 37
JOINT STRAIN AND MALALIGNMENT 44
LIGAMENT INJURIES 47
MUSCULAR STRAINS 48
POSTURAL PAIN 50
VIOLENT INJURY TO THE SPINE 52
SPONDYLOLISTHESIS/SPONDYLOLYSIS 54
STRUCTURAL DEFECTS 55
THE AGEING SPINE 58
CENTRAL CANAL STENOSIS 61
INFLAMMATION AND DISEASE 63

5 ▤ Coping with an acute attack 66
WHEN TO CONSULT YOUR DOCTOR 66
REST AND RELAXATION 67
PAIN RELIEF 70
DAY-TO-DAY LIVING 72

6 ■ A professional diagnosis 74
CONSULTING YOUR DOCTOR 75
CONSULTING A SPECIALIST 77

7 ■ Physiotherapy 82
CONSULTING A PHYSIOTHERAPIST 82
ELECTRONIC EQUIPMENT 84
TRACTION 85
COLLARS AND CORSETS 88
OTHER TREATMENTS 90

8 ■ Manipulation 92
OSTEOPATHY AND CHIROPRACTIC 92
CAN MANIPULATION RELIEVE PAIN? 94
CONDITIONS THAT MAY RESPOND 94
THREE APPROACHES TO BACK PAIN 96

9 ■ Drugs and injections 101
TREATMENT WITH DRUGS 101
INJECTIONS 103

10 ■ Surgery 110
DISCECTOMY 111
DECOMPRESSION 112
SPINAL FUSION 113
SURGERY FOR SCOLIOSIS 115
SURGERY FOR COCCYDINIA 116
SURGERY OF THE NECK 116
FAILURE OF SURGERY 117

11 ■ Acupuncture 118
HEALTH AS HARMONY 118
WILL ACUPUNCTURE HELP? 120
CONSULTING AN ACUPUNCTURIST 121
ALTERNATIVE METHODS 125

12 ■ Alternative therapies 127
HYPNOTHERAPY 127
MEDITATION 129
THE ALEXANDER TECHNIQUE 131

BIOENERGETICS 133
HOMEOPATHY 134
FOOD ALLERGY 135

13 ■ Posture and everyday activities 136
STANDING POSTURE 137
SITTING POSTURE 139
DRIVING 141
LYING DOWN 142
ADAPTING YOUR ENVIRONMENT 144
CARING FOR CHILDREN OR INVALIDS 149
SEXUAL ACTIVITY 151
SPORTS 152

14 ■ Exercise and massage 154
LOWER BACK EXERCISES 157
THERAPEUTIC NECK EXERCISES 163
ANKYLOSING SPONDYLITIS 164
STRENGTHENING EXERCISES 166
SIMPLE RELAXATION 171
RELAXATION THROUGH MASSAGE 172

15 ■ Understanding and coping with pain 175
PAIN PERCEPTION 175
COPING WITH PAIN 179

Conclusion 186
Useful addresses 187
Index 189
Acknowledgments 192

NOTE

Throughout this book the masculine pronoun 'he' is used when referring to the doctor or patient. This is for convenience and does not reflect a preference for either sex.

Preface

The British Holistic Medical Association was launched in 1983 to address a growing need amongst doctors, medical students, the practitioners of alternative, or complementary medicine and the public. This growing need was best expressed by H.R.H. the Prince of Wales when he spoke to the B.M.A. Conference in 1983. He suggested: *"Human nature is such that we are frequently prevented from seeing that what is taken for today's unorthodoxy is probably to be tomorrow's convention".*

He went on to add: *"The whole imposing edifice of modern medicine, for all its breathtaking successes is like the celebrated Tower of Pisa, slightly off-balance".*

"Balance" is a critical concept in "Holism". This new word is not synonymous with complementary or alternative and it must be stressed that the wholesale application of alternative medicine is not one of the aims of the British Holistic Medical Association. Nor is an unthinking and self-destructive criticism of orthodox medicine appropriate. Holism is about responding to the whole person in his or her environment. It involves actively encouraging a partnership between practitioner and patient and this attitude is of particular relevance to the prevention and treatment of back problems.

Back problems are one of the most common presentations both to the doctor and the osteopath. More working days are lost through back pain than all strikes and go-slows put together. It is not just the pain and disability but the chronic distress that accompanies back problems that can be so overwhelming. Yet there are few conditions where a preventative approach is more applicable. It is clear that orthodox medicine is unable to cope with the demands of patients suffering from back pain and a truly holistic approach is now long overdue. This book lays the groundwork for the medicine of the future – a true marriage between the best of technological medicine and the most appropriate therapies for helping a person regain his or her physical, mental and spiritual well-being.

Dr Patrick C. Pietroni MB BS FRCGP MRCP
Senior Lecturer in General Practice
St. Mary's Hospital Medical School, London

Introduction

Back pain is one of the most common afflictions in the industrialized world: about 80 per cent of the population in developed countries suffer from back-ache at some time in their lives. This book is addressed to all those who have back pain, and to anyone who wishes to take preventive measures to minimize their chances of suffering from a back problem in the future. It may also be of use to therapists who want to know what kind of advice they should give to their patients, or who would like more information on available treatments for back pain.

There are already a great many books about back pain. This one stands out for two reasons. Firstly, it is unusual in its breadth of coverage. Too many books on back pain are written by therapists who have specialized in just one aspect of treatment such as manipulation, physiotherapeutic exercises or surgery. This book takes a look at the whole field: at the best of conventional and complementary medicine, and suggests some self-help methods.

Secondly, this book digs deeper than other books. Not only does it explain the causes of back pain in clear, non-technical terms, it also offers practical advice on how to cope when you have a back problem, gives a thorough assessment of the various therapies available, and describes what to expect when you seek professional help. Back pain is a field where there are many changing theories and differing view points. I have tried to sort out what is hard fact about back pain and its treatment, what is probable, and what is mere speculation about the benefits of therapies.

Your doctor's attitude

This book is intended to reassure you that there are many effective ways of treating back trouble. It ought to encourage you to seek out treatment that works for you. No longer should any back specialist, from whatever branch of medicine, be allowed to get away with such off-hand statements as "nothing can be done", "you have got arthritis – learn to live with it", or "you have non-specific back pain". This is simply another way of saying "I don't know what is wrong with you". Your doctor should be sympathetic, not dismissive, about your pain. You will probably find that he fully appreciates the level of pain you are in, and is conscientious in his care for your health. It is likely, though, that he will be non-committal about the prospects of your recovery. Unfortunately, it is extremely difficult to predict how quickly anyone will recover from backache. If the phrase "such and such treatment may help in this condition" creeps into this book now and again, it is either because there is no hard evidence regarding the success of the treatment, or because the disorder responds so variably to different treatments as to be unpredictable.

But then holistic medicine treats individuals, not conditions, and therefore every case in unique. This principle is a theme which runs through this book.

Holistic medicine

The essence of "whole person", or holistic, medicine is diagnosis and treatment taking into account all the factors affecting a person's health, from physical considerations such as biochemical and mechanical factors, to mental factors including motivation towards recovery and ability to adapt.

Much of this information is probably assessed intuitively. Few practitioners deliberately and consciously attempt to quantify all these factors when treating a patient. The holistic practitioner does, however, aspire to this ideal and the better he is, the more likely you are to benefit from this total approach.

The holistic practitioner never loses sight of his patient as a person: he never isolates symptoms from his patient's general health and mental state. Back trouble is not simply a mechanical fault which has to be fixed. Its treatment involves correct use, good posture, freedom from emotional and physical tension and a healthy mental attitude.

Holistic medicine is not a particular form of treatment, it is defined by the practitioner's attitude to his patient, and can embrace both orthodox Western medicine and alternative therapies. The orthodox practitioner may be convinced that pain-killers, bed rest and muscle relaxants are the most effective way of treating someone with back pain, while at the opposite extreme the African witch doctor is convinced that the exorcism of an evil spirit is required to cure his patient. The former is acting primarily on a mechanical and biochemical understanding and the latter on a spiritual interpretation of the problem. Which is the more holistic? Neither, of course, since they are simply approaching the problem from different, but equally narrow-minded angles. Which of them is more effective? In acute lower back pain I suspect that a controlled trial would reveal little difference. Even in our own European culture not so long ago the Germans referred to acute lower back pain as the "Hexenschuss" which means the "witches' blow".

The treatment, therefore, is not necessarily an indication of whether or not the practitioner is holistic. In other words, the employment of standard pharmacological treatments used by the orthodoxy, as opposed to the alternative medicines used by homeopaths and herbalists, does not necessarily imply a less holistic approach. Nevertheless, practitioners of alternative therapies tend to emphasize a holistic approach, and it may be this that accounts for the growing popularity of alternative medicine over orthodox treatment.

Faith in the therapist

The therapist's attitude to you is only part of the story. Your attitude to the practitioner is probably equally important. If you like and trust your therapist, your chances of a cure are much higher than if you dislike him, or have little faith in his ability.

An elegant piece of research into the success of psychiatric techniques illustrates this point very clearly. Two researchers, Caine and Smail, analyzed the therapeutic approaches of a number of psychiatrists and divided them into two groups. The first group practised a "hard, concretistic" approach to the majority of problems, using drugs and electro-convulsive therapy. The second group of psychiatrists adopted a softer approach: counselling, psychotherapy and the use of the therapeutic milieu such as a residential therapeutic community, and preferred a more egalitarian relationship with their patients.

Caine and Smail also analyzed the personality characteristics of each group of psychiatrists. The first group of psychiatrists were more rigid and more authoritarian in character and high in "tough-mindedness" factors, while the second group were higher in "tender-mindedness" qualities.

The researchers then looked at the patients being treated, and divided them into two groups according to the same personality characteristics, regardless of the kind of mental illness from which they were suffering.

Finally, they evaluated the success of the treatment. The results showed that the patients who improved the most were those treated by the psychiatrist of similar personality to themselves, using the therapeutic approach preferred by the patient. The tender-minded patients preferred and improved more with the "softer" counselling approach, while the tough-minded patients did better with the more rigid forms of therapy.

To summarize, it was the relationship between therapist and patient, not the treatment itself, that determined the patients' improvement. Faith in the therapist, trust in his perception and experience of the world, and compatibility between therapist and patient are the important factors. No single method is the right one.

This principle probably applies as much to medicine for physical disorders as to therapy for mental illnesses: there is no particular method of treatment that works best. If you try one type of therapy and find that it does not help you, try another.

Finding the right treatment
Without doubt, some people will be in a better position than others to find appropriate treatment. Health care facilities are not evenly distributed throughout the country. As a medical student, I was outraged by the inequality of health care, particularly training as I did in the East End of London. It would incense me that perinatal mortality rates could vary from as low as ten per 1,000 up to 20 per 1,000 births, depending on which part of the country the mother

lived in. I now appreciate that life carries no guarantees. Some of you will be lucky enough to live close to excellent centres such as the Centre for Spinal Disorders in Oswestry, Shropshire, or Derby's Back School, or the Comprehensive Spine Management Programme in Oregon, USA. Others may know a good local osteopath. For the majority, though, there may seem to be no good local provision.

The need for information
Whatever the case, I strongly exhort all of you to seek out the help you need. In order to make the right choice, though, you need clear and reliable information. Misinformation may lead many people to suffer unnecessarily long. I will quote my own example. At the age of 17, I injured my back lifting heavy concrete blocks on a building site. My mother fortunately had the foresight to take me to a local osteopath who was blind but had good hands. His six week course of exercises and my perseverence got me better quickly. But for many years I had backache if I stood up for long periods, "the cocktail-party back" syndrome; ward rounds as a medical student could go on for torturous hours. I had read that it was important to maintain a hollow curve in the lower back, and I followed this advice. It was ten years later when I studied orthopaedic medicine that I discovered that this posture could be the cause of my back pain. Once I had learned to reduce this curve, my back pain disappeared.

I hope that this book will prevent others from suffering through lack of information. I hope that it will also encourage you to take responsibility for your own health, both by following the advice on self-help given in this book, and by seeking out a therapy that works for you.

1

Who gets back trouble?

If you have had back trouble, or are in pain right now, you have probably asked the question "Why me?". You may be able to recall some awkward twisting or straining action which sparked off the pain, but perhaps the same movement has not injured your back in the past, and other people may be unharmed by similar activities. The chances are that your back was already in a condition where a relatively minor incident was sufficient to trigger the pain, rather like a frayed rope which is snapped by the slightest tug. Though it is difficult to isolate any particular feature which predisposes people to back trouble, factors such as age, occupation and fitness all play a part.

WHO IS MOST AT RISK?

From the jungle of surveys and statistical reports that have been collected in various parts of the world certain common findings emerge.

Vulnerable age groups
You are most likely to have back trouble between the ages of 30 and 50. Few people under 18 and over 60 years of age are affected. The reason for this is not entirely clear but it is likely to be a combination of factors.

The social and occupational demands of the middle years of life are perhaps more intense. Those in their 30s might be bringing up and handling small children, which may involve more lifting and carrying at home. For those at work, the middle years are usually the most productive, whether it be heavy manual work or a sedentary office job.

At this age many people spend less time in sports or leisure activities which could maintain their general fitness and flexibility. It is also during this period that people tend to gain weight, and in addition there is the accumulated effect of 15 years or so of increased mechanical stress and strain on the spine.

From a physiological point of view, the disc (the cushioned pad between each bony segment of the spine) is most vulnerable between the ages of 30 and 50. Young people have strong, resilient discs, while elderly people's discs have dried out and are composed mostly of inelastic fibre. Between these two stages the disc is at greatest risk of injury.

WHAT IS THE TOLL?

Those who escape back pain altogether are a lucky minority: it is estimated that between 60 and 80 per cent of the population in the average industrialized country suffers from back pain at some time in their lives, and that in half of these, the problem will recur.

Questionnaires reveal that as many as half the people who experience back trouble fail to report the symptoms to their doctor. Most of those who do report back pain are either experiencing their first attack, or are chronic sufferers requiring continual medical help. A family doctor's records do not reflect the number of patients registered with him who experience continuing but not incapacitating symptoms, or who develop a recurrence of the problem for which they were treated previously.

Counting the cost

The incidence of reported back pain varies from country to country, but is uniformly high in the industrialized nations. In the United States and Sweden back pain is the single greatest cause of lost time at work in people under the age of 45. In a study undertaken in the Netherlands in 1982, it was revealed that over 50 per cent of people had experienced low back pain. It recurred in 85 per cent of them, and 30 per cent had problems lasting for three months or longer. This rather contradicts the widely quoted statement that 45 per cent of people with acute low back pain recover spontaneously within two weeks and 90 per cent within four weeks.

In Britain, approximately 33 million working days are lost each year through back trouble. On any given day, one in 200 of the workforce will be off work with back trouble which will last for more than six months. Over 4 per cent of people consulting their family doctor are experiencing back trouble for the first time. Some 5 per cent of all new patients attending hospital are there because of back pain, one in 30 of these (41,000 per year) will be admitted to hospital, and one in 12 of these (3,300 per year) will undergo an operation.

Evolutionary factor

Perhaps the problem lies in the way we live. Our ancestors developed around five million years ago and since then men and women have spent most of their time hunting and gathering food. It has been estimated that this kind of work probably entailed around 50 lifting and carrying movements per day. Since the advent of modern society, we have developed a complex environment which may involve some 5,000 lifting and carrying movements each day. Perhaps our social evolution has somewhat outpaced the biological evolution of our spine.

INCIDENCE OF BACK PAIN

Roughly 30 per cent of the population are currently suffering from back pain, but have not sought medical help.

Approximately 25 per cent of the population go through life without experiencing back pain.

Only a minority experiencing back pain now are receiving treatment for their condition.

About 40 per cent will have, or have had back pain, but are not suffering from it now.

Male or female – the weaker sex?

Women seem to be slightly more prone to back trouble than men. The cause for this is not known, but pregnancy, childbirth and child-rearing may take their toll on the spine (see page 149). However, men take more time off work: 627 days per 1000 males are lost from work annually compared to 347 days per 1000 females, although this may reflect the type of work performed by men. Men are twice as likely to undergo surgery.

Physical shape – height and weight

Surprisingly, very little difference can be found in the incidence of back pain between the short, fat individual and the tall, thin one. Only a few out of the several studies on this aspect of back pain show a slightly greater preponderance of back trouble in tall males. Only one study shows that obese people are more at risk than leaner people.

Posture

Poor posture accounts for a high proportion of back pain. However, when discussing posture it is essential to differentiate between various types of posture, all loosely described as poor, but not all of which can be blamed for backache. When we talk about poor posture, we often really mean inelegant posture – in other words, slouching in a chair or walking with hands in pockets. There is no evidence to suggest that such habits increase the risk of back problems. Certain spinal abnormalities which affect posture, such as scoliosis (see page 55), do not necessarily lead to backache unless the condition produces a very obvious deformity.

However, other types of posture are a major cause of backache. Leaning over a desk or working with your arms raised for a long time, lifting heavy weights while bending from your waist instead of at your knees, sitting in a chair of the wrong height or without adequate back support can all result in back problems. These are discussed in Chapter 13.

Fitness and strength

Research suggests that insufficient exercise increases the risk of back problems. If you are fit, your muscles will be strong and flexible, and you will recover more quickly than an unfit person from any injury or illness. Your bones will be stronger too, and if you remain fit as you grow older, your bones will retain their strength for longer than those of an unfit person. However, certain sports such as golf, bowling and baseball – all of which can involve twisting and straining your back – lead to a higher incidence of back trouble. If you have had back problems and wish to take up a new sport, you should consider whether it could harm your back. Your doctor or a physiotherapist specializing in sports injuries should be able to advise you. Competitive sports induce some people to train so intensively that they develop over-use injuries.

Abdominal muscles are the ones that you use when you perform sit-ups. If they are strong they will help to support the spine by increasing pressure in the abdomen, which reduces stress on the lower spine. If your abdominal muscles are weak, your back has to take more weight. This will make you prone to lower back pain, and strengthening the muscles with sit-ups and other exercises (see pages 167 to 168) could help.

The strength of back muscles, however, does not seem to affect the chances of having back trouble unless you are lifting particularly heavy weights. Most of us have back muscles which are quite adequate to cope with normal activities.

Inflexible hamstrings (the large muscles at the back of the thighs), may predispose people to back pain. These muscles pay out whenever you bend forwards, so that your hips do most of the bending. If your hamstrings are stiff, your back has to curve further, and this will increase the risk of back problems. See pages 161 and 162 for exercises to stretch the hamstrings.

A stiff back may not cause trouble. However, therapies which aim to alleviate back pain through making the back more supple are often successful.

HIGH RISK OCCUPATIONS

Many industrial surveys investigate back trouble amongst the whole work-force, including workers with specific and very different tasks. For example, in the building industry the crane-driver, the crane-watcher and the un-skilled labourer all belong to the same trade but experience widely differing loads on their spines.

The evidence to date shows that workers required to lift heavy weights manually are most at risk, particularly unskilled and older labourers. Each year, about 22 per cent of these people report back trouble, followed by nurses at 17 per cent each year.

Those in sedentary jobs however, are undoubtedly almost as much at risk as manual workers, particularly if the job entails driving long distances. Truck drivers, bus drivers, tractor drivers and aeroplane pilots tend to develop lower back pain at an earlier age and show in-creased X-ray evidence of degenerative disease in the spine. Vibration of the vehicles they drive is probably to blame.

BACK PAIN AT WORK

The incidence of back pain varies according to the occupation, which can be divided into three main categories: heavy, intermediate and light. The sample jobs below are listed within each category in order of decreasing frequency of back trouble.

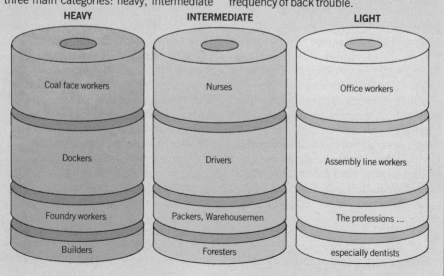

HEAVY	INTERMEDIATE	LIGHT
Coal face workers	Nurses	Office workers
Dockers	Drivers	Assembly line workers
Foundry workers	Packers, Warehousemen	The professions ...
Builders	Foresters	especially dentists

Hazardous activities

All of these factors increase the chances of back problems, however, in many cases the risks can be minimized by learning correct techniques for lifting and carrying, and by using appropriate equipment. See Chapter 13 for further advice on reducing risks.

● Lifting of weights manually
● Bending, twisting and reaching
● Repetitive work with lighter loads
● Static work postures – for example, driving, assembling electronic parts, sewing, weaving
● Vibration – as in driving a tractor
● Monotony and work dissatisfaction (increases absenteeism rate)
● Stooping and prolonged bending
● Lifting very heavy weights suddenly
● Lifting an unexpectedly light weight.

Risk factors at work

● Unacceptable workloads (recommendations such as a maximum of half body weight for occasional handling, and 40 per cent of body weight for continuous lifting, were made as early as 1927)
● Rapid, repetitive handling tasks
● Inappropriate working heights
● Poor seating without back rest, arm supports, or swivel action
● Inadequate working space within which to turn or move
● Poor viewing distance for sedentary workers
● Tools/controls not within easy reach.

PSYCHOLOGICAL FACTORS

During the last years of his life, Louis Pasteur, the father of modern microbiology, said that if he could start again, instead of looking at how the microbe invaded its host, he would want to know what it was about a particular host that was so attractive. In other words, why do we sometimes catch every bug that is going round while at other times we can be surrounded by friends and relatives who have all been stricken and yet we remain apparently immune? You may ask much the same question if you have back pain. It may well be that you are at a high risk age and in a high risk profession as far as back pain is concerned, but you probably have colleagues of a similar age who have never felt so much as a twinge in the back.

No-one can say for certain why some people are prone to back pain, while others who have a similar physique and live in similar circumstances are not, but the answer seems to lie partly in emotional or psychological factors.

We accept that there are many everyday examples of physical reactions governed by the emotions – blushing, fainting at the sight of blood or the desire to defaecate when struck by panic – and it may well be that some people develop backache by similar mechanisms. On many occasions patients admit that they have been under a lot of stress and ask "Do you think that it has anything to do with my back pain?" To me it seems no more than common sense to appreciate that continuous emotional or psychological stress can produce functional changes in the body, which become structural if they are perpetuated.

I have come across numerous cases of back pain where there is a psychological or emotional element. Muscular tension resulting from suppressed emotions is frequently a cause of neck pain and headaches as well as back pain.

The two cases cited opposite demonstrate how stress can produce severe acute or chronic back problems.

CASE HISTORIES

Physical and mental tension can often be blamed for precipitating back problems, as the following case histories show. The first patient was suffering from a physical injury caused, at least in part, by his mental state. The symptoms of the second patient, though, may have originated entirely in emotional tension.

Acute disc prolapse

The patient was a 40-year-old man who developed acute low back pain after helping his neighbours to unload some carpet from a van. It was a typical case of acute disc prolapse (see page 37). At first impression it looked like simple cause and effect, but the three other men who had been with him were uninjured, even though all four were of similar strength and all in sedentary occupations. To understand the problem, it is necessary to look further than the simple physical activity which triggered the pain. It transpired that this particular man had been working up to 16 hours a day in a hostel for maladjusted teenagers, commuting an hour or so by car to work and back, sitting in meetings for hours at a time and worrying about the teenagers under his care.

The man was already mentally and emotionally drained and physically unfit. He was very tense and under stress, so out of the four men, he was the one to succumb to back pain. To prevent a recurrence of this problem, he needed to make a constructive review of his workload, emotional stress and physical activities, and to get himself fitter as well as to learn correct techniques for lifting and handling heavy objects.

Chronic back pain

One young woman came to me with a multitude of symptoms affecting her whole back, neck and shoulders, with disturbed sensations in her arms and pain even into her buttocks and legs. Over the previous years these had come and gone, irregularly and inexplicably, with varying severity. She had consulted other doctors about her symptoms before coming to my surgery. On examination there was no identifiable structural problem in the spine or in any other joints, but there was a fair amount of tension in the muscles.

The key to diagnosing her problem lay in understanding the reasons for this excessive tension. Her background history revealed that she had lost her father in her mid teens and apparently never reacted in the usual way by grieving. Two or three years later she became pregnant while unmarried and was persuaded by her mother to have the baby adopted. Over the following year or two, she developed the set of symptoms already described, and was investigated medically and diagnosed as suffering from multiple sclerosis. Shortly after this, she married and became pregnant again. On medical advice, both she and her husband agreed to have the pregnancy terminated. Presumably it was thought that she would not be able to cope with the baby in the future if her medical condition deteriorated.

All this emerged whilst I was examining the muscles by hand and providing a gentle but deep massage. As her story poured out so also did her feelings about the past and her fear of the label multiple sclerosis. A week later she reported that 90 per cent of her chronic symptoms had disappeared. After one or two more treatment sessions, mostly one spent in counselling, with some simple massage, it became more evident both to her and myself that her body had manifested the suppressed grief of three major traumas in a set of symptoms that had been mislabelled by the medical profession. Consequently, she began to feel that it was extremely unlikely that she had ever suffered from multiple sclerosis in the first place, which was another fear dispelled.

YOUR OWN BACK PAIN

Certain common phrases in everyday language have probably developed from an instinctive understanding of psycho-somatic problems. You might ask yourself the following questions:

● I have a pain in the neck – Who is a pain in the neck?

● My muscles feel tight – What is making me uptight?

● Is anyone giving me the hump?

● I can't straighten up – Am I stooping too low (to take on that job, to accept that kind of money)?

● I feel a weight across my shoulders – What is the cross I have to bear?

There are numerous other colloquialisms, which express the language of our bodies. Try applying some of these to your own predicament and see what comes up – you may be surprised.

Fluctuating moods

Even your day-to-day mood can affect the incidence of back trouble. Many people notice that on some days they can dig the garden or do the housework without irritating their backs, while on other days their backs will ache at the slightest excuse. It seems likely that emotional moods can affect the state of your back just as much as the physical factors which we generally associate with such problems. Consider how often your posture reflects your mood. When you are feeling low and depressed your head will tend to hang low and your shoulders will hunch. If you are feeling resigned and defeatist, you will probably slouch more. When you are feeling angry or irritable, you will be more careless as to how you use your back in bending and lifting.

Spend a few days observing how your mood affects your posture and how you use your back. Notice that when you are feeling buoyant, proud and happy, your back very rarely seems to play up or at the very most, you feel only an occasional twinge. Whenever there is psychological disharmony the chances are that there will also be physical dysfunction. As you become more aware of how your emotional state affects your posture, you may be able to avert back trouble by taking extra care and perhaps resolving the inner conflict if at all possible.

It is all too easy to blame external circumstances, especially when we are suppressing anger and resentment. An awkward movement may just be "the straw that breaks the camel's back", while the emotional tension is the predisposing factor.

Stress: spinal and emotional

Many people are under constant pressure for long periods, without time for adequate rest or holidays. They have lost touch with the needs of their own bodies, the need for adequate recreation physically, for relaxation and sleep. I find that many business people in particular who have developed acute back pain are under stress from high overheads, meeting deadlines for delivery, jet travel, or simply striving to succeed in a highly competitive field. The 30-50 year old man is at great risk and often he is driving himself mentally far harder than his emotional or physical system can cope with. Back pain is the body's way of protesting against stress and enforcing a general slowing down. I often advise such patients to take several days off work, to re-order and balance their lives, or to rest and to use this time productively to re-assess their priorities. Not only does this period of rest help the bout of acute pain, but it also helps to guard against a recurrence.

2
The healthy back

The spine is a superb and fascinating piece of engineering. It is the central support system for the entire body and is used in almost all our movements. In addition, it supports and protects the spinal cord – a rope-like bundle of nerve fibres which relays messages from the brain to all parts of the body.

The function and structure of the spine are virtually identical in all mammals. However, our upright posture has created a few differences. When mammals evolved from swinging in the trees to walking on all fours on the ground, they no longer needed a tail for counterbalance. Instead, their centre of gravity shifted to the point between their front and rear limbs. Then as they learned to walk on their hind legs, leaving their forelimbs free to grasp and hold on to objects, their spines needed to change shape yet again. The forces of gravity exerted on an upright human are pulling vertically through the length of the body, so the human spine became a vertical shock absorber, with curvatures to provide the necessary resilience.

Development of the spine

The spine is not just a rigid support system: its structure is essential to walking and many other movements. We walk not only with our legs, but with our whole back, and we reach for, grasp and carry objects not just with our arms but also with our back. Consider our origins among the fishes and amphibians, long before the development of the primates, and then look at the way a fish moves in the water: its propulsion comes not from the fins but from flowing movements of the spine controlled by the longitudinal muscles which move the tail from side to side. The fins are there largely for stability and direction. Even though our form has changed over the millennia, the basic structure of the spine has not, and in the foreseeable future will not lose its function in locomotion.

THE SPINE

The spine is a column consisting of up to 34 bones, running from the base of the skull all the way down the back. There are 24 individual bony segments called vertebrae. The "tail-bone" consists of five fused segments called the sacrum, which adjoins one hip bone on each side to make up the pelvis. Below this we have between three and five (strangely enough, the number varies but most of us have four) fused or partially mobile segments which form the coccyx, the rudimentary tail that is our primate inheritance.

THE SPINAL COLUMN

The column of bones that makes up the spinal column is the central support for the skeleton, the scaffold that supports the body and protects the organs. The skull, which contains the brain, is supported chiefly by the first two cervical vertebrae. The thoracic vertebrae are each joined to a rib on either side — the cage formed by the ribs is the frame that surrounds and protects the organs such as the heart, lungs and liver.

The basin formed by the sacrum and the two hip bones — the pelvis — protects the organs of the lower body, the bladder and the reproductive organs.

The spine is a very mobile structure; it can bend and rotate in almost any direction. The most mobile regions are the cervical (neck) and lumbar (lower back) regions — movement in all directions in the thoracic region is restricted by the rib-cage.

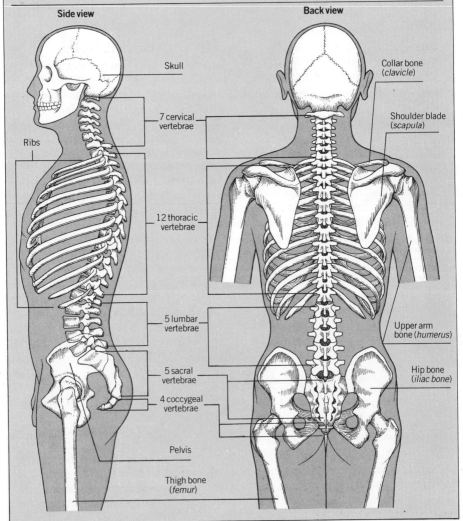

Side view

Skull

7 cervical vertebrae

Ribs

12 thoracic vertebrae

5 lumbar vertebrae

5 sacral vertebrae

4 coccygeal vertebrae

Pelvis

Thigh bone (*femur*)

Back view

Collar bone (*clavicle*)

Shoulder blade (*scapula*)

Upper arm bone (*humerus*)

Hip bone (*iliac bone*)

The 24 movable vertebrae above the sacrum are divided into three groups: 7 cervical (neck), 12 thoracic (chest) and 5 lumbar (lower back).

The vertebrae

The main part of a vertebrae is more or less cylindrical, with flat surfaces at the top and bottom. To the back of this main section of the vertebra is a hole, and when the vertebrae are stacked up, these holes form a continuous channel – the spinal or neural canal – which contains the spinal cord (see page 21).

Behind the spinal canal each vertebra has seven projections, known as processes. They form three pairs and an odd one out, the spinous process. The spinous processes are the knobbly bits which you can feel down your back.

The remaining pairs of processes lie to the right and left of this. Two of these pairs – the upper articular processes and the lower articular processes – act as joints to link the vertebrae together and strengthen the spine. The back muscles are attached to the remaining pair, the transverse processes, and the spinous process, which provide anchorage as the muscles contract and relax.

Facet joints

The upper articular processes of one vertebra link up to the lower articular

---

THE VERTEBRAE

No two vertebrae are exactly alike but there are definite groups. Shown here are the last two thoracic vertebrae and the first two lumbar vertebrae. The spinous processes are much larger in the lumbar vertebrae, and the thoracic vertebrae have small flat areas, costal facets, on the side where they are attached to the ribs.

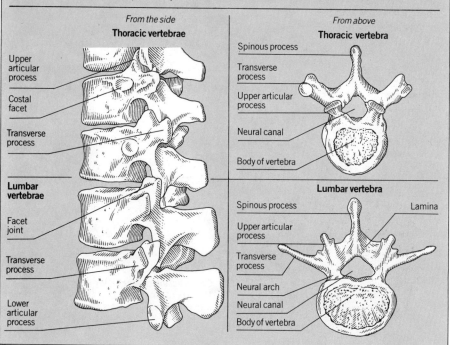

From the side
Thoracic vertebrae

Upper articular process

Costal facet

Transverse process

Lumbar vertebrae

Facet joint

Transverse process

Lower articular process

From above
Thoracic vertebra

Spinous process

Transverse process

Upper articular process

Neural canal

Body of vertebra

Lumbar vertebra

Spinous process

Lamina

Upper articular process

Transverse process

Neural arch

Neural canal

Body of vertebra

processes of the vertebra above. These processes have flat smooth surfaces like the facets of a diamond, hence the name facet joints. They are also known as apophyseal joints or posterior joints.

The articulating surfaces of these joints are lined with cartilage, and lubricated with a special fluid (synovial fluid), the whole joint being contained within a capsule. Movement of a regular and repetitive kind is essential for healthy cartilage and helps to keep the joints working efficiently.

Discs

The flat surface on the top and bottom of the main body of the vertebra is covered in a thin layer of cartilage called an end plate. Each vertebra is further separated by a cartilage pad known as a disc. The outer layers, called the annulus fibrosus, are formed from tough fibrous cartilage. The inner part of the disc is a semi-fluid, gel-like substance, and is known as the nucleus pulposus. This gel allows the disc to mould itself like a liquid ball-bearing, so that in addition to acting as a joint, the disc performs a second equally vital function as a cushion between each vertebra. The annulus fibrosus also blends with the cartilage on the surface of the vertebrae.

The disc is largely composed of water – 90 per cent in babies and still 70 per

---

SPINAL JOINTS

The joints between the vertebrae are made up of several different elements. A disc separates the main body of each vertebra and works like a ball-bearing to allow the spine to twist and bend (see opposite) and to act as a shock absorber. The facet joints of the articular processes form a fulcrum, allowing a pincer movement to be made by the spinal joints when the spine bends backwards or forwards.

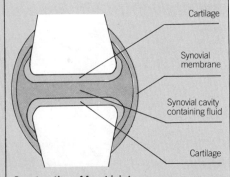

Disc acting as shock absorber

Body of vertebra

Facet joint acting as fulcrum

Ligament

Construction of a disc
The annulus fibrosus is made up of layers of concentric fibres that cross each other obliquely on the outer edge, becoming more upright as they near the centre. The nucleus pulposus is made of a gelatinous substance.

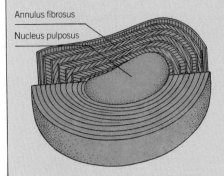

Annulus fibrosus

Nucleus pulposus

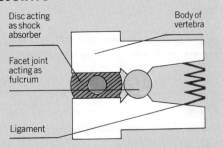

Cartilage

Synovial membrane

Synovial cavity containing fluid

Cartilage

Construction of facet joint
The articulating surfaces of the joint are covered with cartilage. The joint is surrounded by a membrane which secretes a fluid that lubricates the joint.

cent in a 70-year-old. Exercise of a repetitive kind, provided that it is not excessive, encourages a good balance of fluid as opposed to fibre, and helps to keep drying out and degeneration at bay. Similarly, the discs need adequate periods of rest from the weight of the upper body pressing down – a disc can shrink by 10 per cent of its height during the day, which is why you are slightly taller in the morning than in the evening – as much as 2 cm overall. A night's rest enables the disc to reabsorb nutrition and fluid, which allows it to regain the height lost over the day.

The healthy disc is extremely strong: it has to be in order to absorb shocks. When compressed (it has a breaking strength of 800kg in the young and 450kg in the elderly) it is stronger than the bone of a vertebra. It is, however, more susceptible to stresses caused by twisting motions, and the outer layers can rupture.

The disc cartilage contains a few pain-sensitive nerves, but the pain associated with a so-called slipped disc (a misnomer, since a disc cannot slip) often comes from an injured disc pressing on the dural sheath or a nerve.

The disc has no blood supply and derives its nutrition by absorbing nutrients

How the disc allows movement
If you think of the vertebrae as two pieces of wood and the nucleus pulposus as a soft rubber ball-bearing, as shown, it is easy to see why the disc forms such a mobile joint.

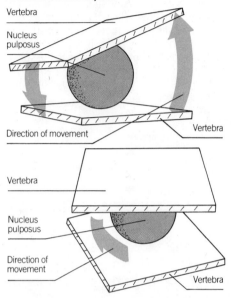

Vertebra

Nucleus pulposus

Direction of movement

Vertebra

Vertebra

Nucleus pulposus

Direction of movement

Vertebra

through the small areas of cartilage, the end-plates, of the adjacent vertebrae. Providing that the nucleus is intact and the outer layers are undamaged, the disc can absorb compressive and jarring forces very efficiently, distributing loading forces by adapting its shape.

THE SPINAL CANAL

The vertebrae provide a continuous channel called the spinal canal, down which the spinal cord runs. The spinal cord is a bundle of nerves which connects the brain with nerves throughout the body, relaying information to the brain, and messages from the brain to other parts of the body. It runs from the base of the skull down to the lumbar vertebrae. Below this, the nerves run out in strands which, owing to their

appearance, have been given the name *cauda equina*, meaning horse's tail.

At regular intervals, pairs of spinal nerves branch off through foramina (gaps in the vertebral column) then divide up to send nerves to the rest of the body. The spinal cord is surrounded by three membranes, which are called meninges. The outermost layer is a sheath or tube called the dura, which runs down as far as the second of the five fused bones

THE SPINAL CORD

The spinal cord provides the vital link between the brain and the nerves in the rest of the body. It is continuous with the brain stem, and finishes at the first or second lumbar vertebra. It is surrounded and protected by the same three membranes that protect the brain. Damage to the spinal cord can result in temporary or permanent disorders of any part of the body below the site of injury.

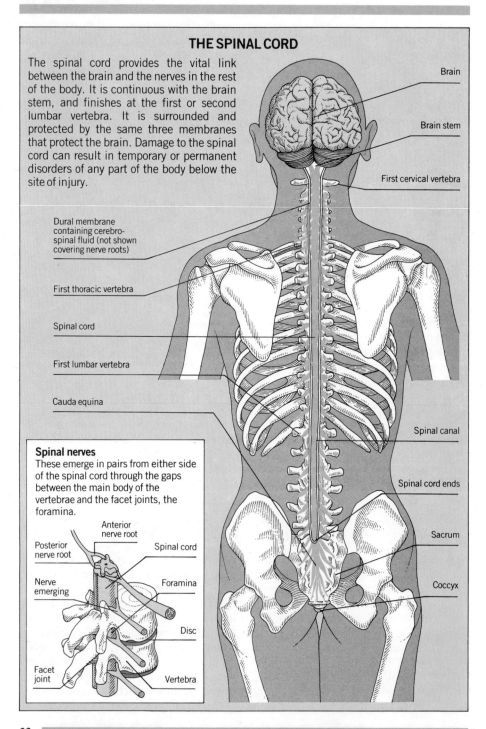

Brain

Brain stem

First cervical vertebra

Dural membrane containing cerebro-spinal fluid (not shown covering nerve roots)

First thoracic vertebra

Spinal cord

First lumbar vertebra

Cauda equina

Spinal canal

Spinal cord ends

Sacrum

Coccyx

Spinal nerves

These emerge in pairs from either side of the spinal cord through the gaps between the main body of the vertebrae and the facet joints, the foramina.

Anterior nerve root

Posterior nerve root

Spinal cord

Nerve emerging

Foramina

Disc

Facet joint

Vertebra

which form the sacrum. At the points where the pairs of nerve roots emerge from the spinal cord through the foramina, pairs of dural root sleeves project from the dura to enclose and protect them.

The dural sheath is extremely responsive to pressure and is mobile throughout its length up to the point at which it is attached to the sacrum. The dural sheath and root sleeves are slightly flexible, but certain movements can cause the nerve to rub against the vertebra, which explains why stretching the nerve in the leg raising test can cause pain in some people (see page 76).

Inside the sheath, between the two inner layers, is the cerebro-spinal fluid which bathes the spinal cord and is continuous with the fluid surrounding the brain. It acts as an extra shock absorber to protect the sensitive spinal cord. The dural sheath forms a barrier maintaining the particular chemical environment which is essential to the cells of the central nervous system.

LIGAMENTS AND MUSCLES

Superimposed on the basic skeletal structure of the spine are the ligaments and muscles. Both are involved in movement of the joints.

THE LIGAMENTS
Joints are supported by tough, inelastic bands of fibre, the ligaments. These help to hold the bones together firmly and strengthen the small joints at each segment. In combination with the facet joints, they keep the spine in one piece, allowing only a limited range of movement in any one direction, according to their length.

The main ligaments run down the length of the spine at the back and front, while others bind and strengthen the joints. The ligaments require regular movement otherwise they will eventually become stiff or slack. Once this has happened, whether through ageing, disuse, or scarring, it is difficult to restore them to their original condition, so it is most important to ensure that they receive sufficient exercise.

THE MUSCLES
Around each joint there is a group of muscles. Each end of a muscle is firmly

Spinal ligaments
A complicated network of ligaments holds all the spinal joints together. The ligaments around the main body of the vertebrae, the anterior and posterior ligaments, extend right round the column to support it.

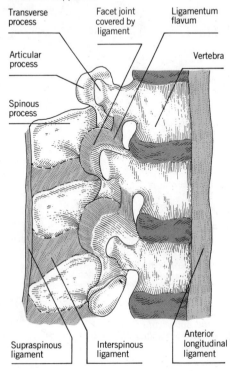

Transverse process

Articular process

Spinous process

Facet joint covered by ligament

Ligamentum flavum

Vertebra

Supraspinous ligament

Interspinous ligament

Anterior longitudinal ligament

THE MUSCLES OF THE BACK

This diagram will give you an idea of how the layers of muscle are built up. The right side of the body shows the small muscles, those mainly concerned with postural adjustment; the left side shows how the larger muscles involved in movement are laid over the top.

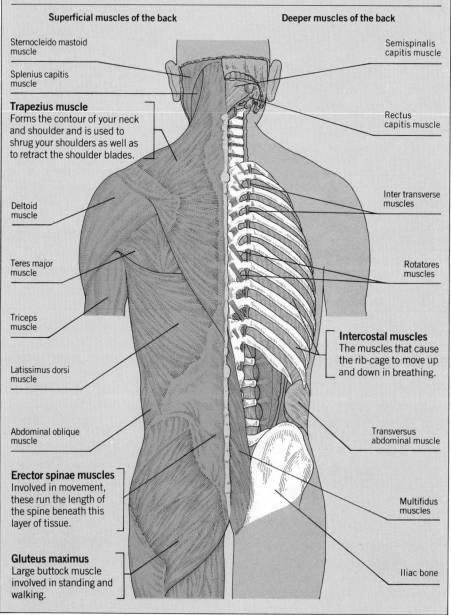

Superficial muscles of the back

Sternocleido mastoid muscle

Splenius capitis muscle

Trapezius muscle
Forms the contour of your neck and shoulder and is used to shrug your shoulders as well as to retract the shoulder blades.

Deltoid muscle

Teres major muscle

Triceps muscle

Latissimus dorsi muscle

Abdominal oblique muscle

Erector spinae muscles
Involved in movement, these run the length of the spine beneath this layer of tissue.

Gluteus maximus
Large buttock muscle involved in standing and walking.

Deeper muscles of the back

Semispinalis capitis muscle

Rectus capitis muscle

Inter transverse muscles

Rotatores muscles

Intercostal muscles
The muscles that cause the rib-cage to move up and down in breathing.

Transversus abdominal muscle

Multifidus muscles

Iliac bone

attached to a different bone, either directly or by means of a band of tissue known as a tendon. The muscles are made up of bundles of fibres that receive messages from the brain which cause them to contract, resulting in movement of the joint. Muscles tend to work in pairs: when one muscle contracts, the opposite one relaxes. They vary in their main function and the back muscles fall into several groups.

Close to the joints of the vertebrae are multitudes of small muscles which can provide subtle alterations of movement by means of small contractions. These muscles are mainly for providing posture control.

The large muscles

More superficially visible in a lean person are the longer, larger and stronger muscles which control the major movements of the trunk. At the back, these are the muscles known as the erector spinae (literally, "spine raisers"). These pay out when you bend over, resisting the force of gravity, and have to contract even more strongly when you straighten up, thereby exerting great compressive force on the spine.

Across the front of the body and at the sides, the abdominal muscles play an important part in helping to support the spine by maintaining pressure inside the abdomen and chest. This pressure provides an essential measure of counter-support to the spine especially when you lift something. You can see a good example of this when you watch a professional weightlifter holding his breath and tensing his abdominal muscles in order to lift a large weight.

How the muscles move the trunk

When you twist or rotate your spine, the abdominal muscles and the back muscles play an important role. Think

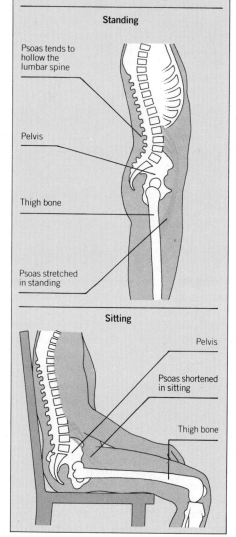

PSOAS MUSCLES

A large group of muscles in the abdomen, the psoas are attached at one end to the transverse processes of the lumbar vertebrae, and are anchored at the other end on the upper part of the thigh bone. They are involved in flexing the hips, for walking or climbing stairs, for example, and play an important role in maintaining posture for sitting and standing.

Standing

Psoas tends to hollow the lumbar spine

Pelvis

Thigh bone

Psoas stretched in standing

Sitting

Pelvis

Psoas shortened in sitting

Thigh bone

of the golf player who needs to create a strong twisting force to effect a good drive. This has to be balanced by an equal and opposite twisting movement which is transmitted through the spine and the lower limbs. For example, try standing on a platform and swinging a golf club – the balancing force created by the opposing muscles makes the platform rotate in the opposite direction.

Superimposed over the back muscles are the muscles that control and move the shoulder girdle in the upper back and the hip girdle in the lower back. The muscles supporting your hip joints are very large and strong and form the contours of the buttock and hip. The deeper layers of muscles are smaller and exert a rotating force on your hip joints.

Maintaining healthy muscles

Muscles have to be able to contract and shorten – some muscles contract to one third of their original length. When relaxed, they can also be stretched and they are therefore to some extent elastic. If your muscles are to be maintained at the peak of performance, they must have a good supply of blood and energy. All living tissue requires oxygen and nutrients to stay alive, and if the blood supply to your muscles is reduced – perhaps because a muscle has gone into protective spasm in reaction to pain (see page 68), or has become chronically contracted due to poor posture – then the cells and tissues will suffer and their function will be impaired. If this state of affairs continues for long enough, the muscle or muscles will become painful, weak or less elastic, and will eventually shorten. Like ligaments, muscles also need regular work in the form of contractions if they are to maintain their strength and encourage healthy local circulation. Muscles that have been contracted for long periods to maintain a

HOW NERVES STIMULATE MUSCLES

HOW NERVES STIMULATE MUSCLES

The nervous system is made up of millions of nerve fibres. These fibres transmit electrical impulses to and from the brain, connecting the brain with the rest of the body. The nerves are divided into two types: sensory fibres, which send signals, such as pain messages, to the brain; and motor fibres, which relay messages from the brain to the muscles. Muscles consist of bundles of fibres that are controlled by impulses from the nerves.

When you decide to bend your arm, for example, the brain sends out a message which is transmitted along the appropriate nerves to your biceps, the muscle in the upper arm. This signal makes the biceps contract, which pulls your forearm up, bending your arm at the elbow.

certain posture – for example, if you have been sitting writing or typing – need regular stretching to prevent them becoming shorter and weaker.

In addition, because muscles are controlled by nerves (see above), excessive nervous system stimulation, such as might be caused by pain from an injury or even simply by tension, can make the muscles tense up. Relaxation is therefore another important ingredient in the recipe for healthy muscles.

Finally, an intact nerve supply is essential to healthy muscles because no muscle can move unless it receives the correct signals from its corresponding nerve. In fact the nerve, its signals and the muscle fibre act as one unit – the motor unit. If, as a result of an injury or an infection, a nerve is severed or its cell unit in the spinal cord is damaged, the muscle cannot contract and will waste away. An example of this is found in poliomyelitis, in which a virus damages the cells in the spinal cord, resulting in permanent weakness in certain muscles.

FUNCTIONS OF THE SPINE

In order to understand how all these separate parts of the back interrelate, it is useful to think of each area of the spine in relation to its functions.

Your neck must be strong enough to hold your head, which is a considerable weight – an adult's head can weigh as much as 6-9 kg (14-20 lb). It must also be sufficiently flexible to allow you to turn your head for looking and listening. At the same time, you must be able to maintain a level gaze and not upset your organs of balance, which are located deep in the outer ear and are finely tuned to the gravitational and rotational forces. We all tend to rely on a level gaze as a matter of course, but think of a hand-held cine camera and the way that the picture goes to pieces if the holder suddenly has to run – yet that same person will generally be able to see what is happening as he or she moves, with no difficulty at all. We achieve this steady gaze through complex feedback mechanisms in the neck and the organs of balance in the ears, which allow the brain to account for movement when interpreting visual information.

Movement in the mid back

The thorax or chest, which includes the ribs, allows the movement entailed in drawing breath. When you inhale fully, the thoracic spine extends slightly as the ribs rise, and when you exhale, the thoracic spine flexes.

Movement in the lower back

The lumbar region lies below the thoracic part of the spine and must be solid and very strong to support the weight of the upper half of your body. It must also be flexible so that you can bend and reach the ground. Bending forwards from the thoracic spine is more limited because it would restrict your capacity to breathe by preventing expansion of the lungs.

The pelvis, including the five fused vertebrae of the sacrum, must provide a firm base for your abdomen. The pelvis transmits the forces from your spine to your legs through your hip joints and your sacroiliac joints (the strong joints between the sacrum and the ilium). This downwards force counteracts the shock wave which comes up from each foot and leg when you walk or run and which is transmitted through the hip joint and sacroiliac joint into the spine. Some of this force is counterbalanced across the pubic arch of the pelvis, but this whole area must withstand these frequent shearing, or asymmetrical forces, reducing the load on the spine.

The importance of a healthy back

Your spine, therefore, has to be firm enough to support the body weight in standing erect, but at the same time it must be strong and flexible enough to provide a firm anchorage and the source of movement of the upper and lower limbs. In addition it must provide a safe, cushioned channel for nerves. In order to achieve this, all the separate parts of the spine – bones and joints, discs, ligaments, muscles and nervous system – must be working in unison, each one making its contribution of stability, power, movement, strength or flexibility. Most of the time we walk, stretch, lift, carry, make love or drive a car without having to worry about our backs, and it is worth remembering, if you are suffering from back pain, that most back sufferers – given a little patience, common sense self-help and the right treatment – can return to the happy state of relying on a healthy back.

3

Making your own diagnosis

There are many different causes of back pain. Almost any segment of the spine can be damaged and give rise to pain. Disorders of other parts of the body, particularly the lungs, kidneys and female reproductive organs can also cause backache. This book deals almost exclusively with spinal causes of back pain.

Most back pain is neither severe nor serious, and can be treated adequately at home. However, since pain anywhere in the back can be a symptom of a serious disorder, it is important that you have some idea of what might be causing your pain, so that you can decide what action to take.

This chapter will help you to make that decision, and will direct you to the sections in the rest of the book that are relevant to your disorder. Use whichever chart deals with the area of your pain, or with the part of your back that is most painful. If your entire back is painful and other areas of your body ache and you have a fever, you probably have flu, a cause of back pain which is not covered in detail in this book.

Start with the question at the top of the relevant chart, and answer either "yes" or "no". Pain counts as starting suddenly if it builds up over no more than a few hours, perhaps overnight.

This will lead you to your next question; progress through the chart in this way until you reach a diagnosis box. This is just a very tentative diagnosis; only a doctor will be able to give a firm diagnosis of your symptoms. However, it will give you an idea of what might be the cause of your pain, and offer some advice on what you should do. If none of the diagnoses fit your symptoms, you should see your doctor to find out what is wrong. It does not necessarily mean that none of the disorders here is causing your pain, since symptoms vary greatly. This flowchart covers only the most common patterns of symptoms.

Where the chart indicates that you must seek urgent medical help, call your doctor immediately or go to your nearest casualty department without delay. When it suggests that you should see your doctor, this is not an emergency, but you should consult your doctor within the next few days. Where there is no advice to contact your doctor, see the appropriate section in the next chapter, which outlines the nature of the disorder that is most likely to be causing your pain, and gives more detailed advice on how you should cope. You may still, of course, want medical help, particularly if your pain is severe.

LOWER BACK OR LEG PAIN

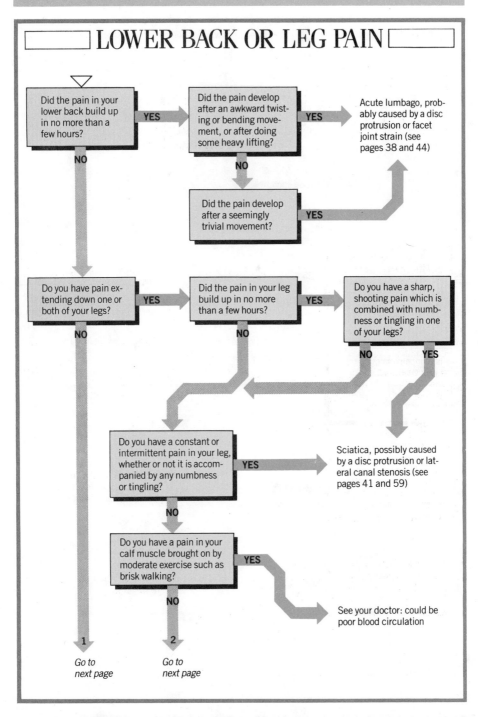

Did the pain in your lower back build up in no more than a few hours? **YES** → Did the pain develop after an awkward twisting or bending movement, or after doing some heavy lifting? **YES** → Acute lumbago, probably caused by a disc protrusion or facet joint strain (see pages 38 and 44)

NO

Did the pain develop after a seemingly trivial movement? **YES** →

Do you have pain extending down one or both of your legs? **YES** → Did the pain in your leg build up in no more than a few hours? **YES** → Do you have a sharp, shooting pain which is combined with numbness or tingling in one of your legs?

NO — **NO** — **NO** **YES**

Do you have a constant or intermittent pain in your leg, whether or not it is accompanied by any numbness or tingling? **YES** → Sciatica, possibly caused by a disc protrusion or lateral canal stenosis (see pages 41 and 59)

NO

Do you have a pain in your calf muscle brought on by moderate exercise such as brisk walking? **YES** → See your doctor: could be poor blood circulation

NO

1
Go to
next page

2
Go to
next page

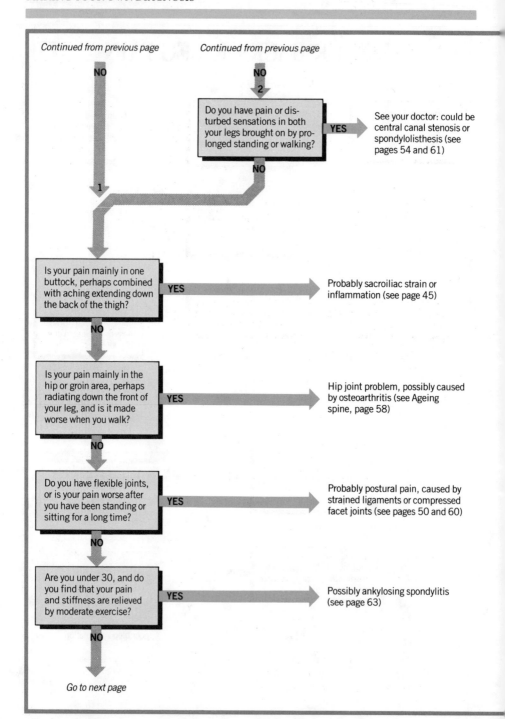

Continued from previous page

Continued from previous page

NO

NO
2

Do you have pain or disturbed sensations in both your legs brought on by prolonged standing or walking? **YES** → See your doctor: could be central canal stenosis or spondylolisthesis (see pages 54 and 61)

NO

1

Is your pain mainly in one buttock, perhaps combined with aching extending down the back of the thigh? **YES** → Probably sacroiliac strain or inflammation (see page 45)

NO

Is your pain mainly in the hip or groin area, perhaps radiating down the front of your leg, and is it made worse when you walk? **YES** → Hip joint problem, possibly caused by osteoarthritis (see Ageing spine, page 58)

NO

Do you have flexible joints, or is your pain worse after you have been standing or sitting for a long time? **YES** → Probably postural pain, caused by strained ligaments or compressed facet joints (see pages 50 and 60)

NO

Are you under 30, and do you find that your pain and stiffness are relieved by moderate exercise? **YES** → Possibly ankylosing spondylitis (see page 63)

NO

Go to next page

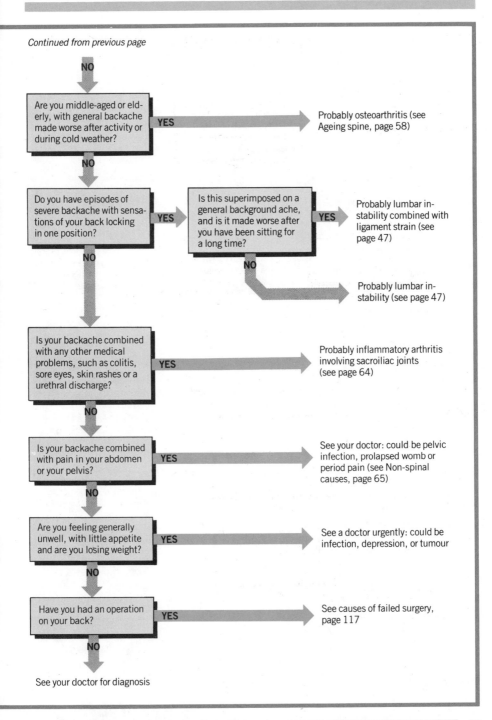

Continued from previous page

NO

Are you middle-aged or elderly, with general backache made worse after activity or during cold weather? — **YES** → Probably osteoarthritis (see Ageing spine, page 58)

NO

Do you have episodes of severe backache with sensations of your back locking in one position? — **YES** → Is this superimposed on a general background ache, and is it made worse after you have been sitting for a long time? — **YES** → Probably lumbar instability combined with ligament strain (see page 47)

NO → Probably lumbar instability (see page 47)

NO

Is your backache combined with any other medical problems, such as colitis, sore eyes, skin rashes or a urethral discharge? — **YES** → Probably inflammatory arthritis involving sacroiliac joints (see page 64)

NO

Is your backache combined with pain in your abdomen or your pelvis? — **YES** → See your doctor: could be pelvic infection, prolapsed womb or period pain (see Non-spinal causes, page 65)

NO

Are you feeling generally unwell, with little appetite and are you losing weight? — **YES** → See a doctor urgently: could be infection, depression, or tumour

NO

Have you had an operation on your back? — **YES** → See causes of failed surgery, page 117

NO

See your doctor for diagnosis

MID BACK PAIN

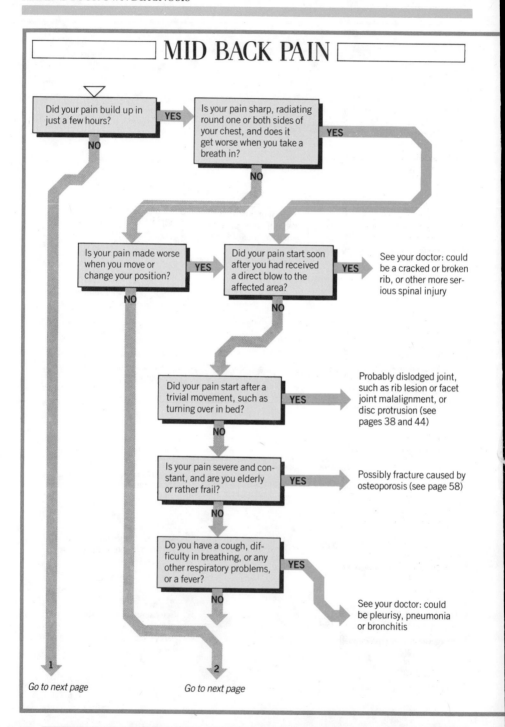

Did your pain build up in just a few hours?

YES → Is your pain sharp, radiating round one or both sides of your chest, and does it get worse when you take a breath in?

YES → See your doctor: could be a cracked or broken rib, or other more serious spinal injury

NO

NO

Is your pain made worse when you move or change your position?

YES → Did your pain start soon after you had received a direct blow to the affected area?

YES → See your doctor: could be a cracked or broken rib, or other more serious spinal injury

NO

NO

Did your pain start after a trivial movement, such as turning over in bed?

YES → Probably dislodged joint, such as rib lesion or facet joint malalignment, or disc protrusion (see pages 38 and 44)

NO

Is your pain severe and constant, and are you elderly or rather frail?

YES → Possibly fracture caused by osteoporosis (see page 58)

NO

Do you have a cough, difficulty in breathing, or any other respiratory problems, or a fever?

YES → See your doctor: could be pleurisy, pneumonia or bronchitis

NO

1
Go to next page

2
Go to next page

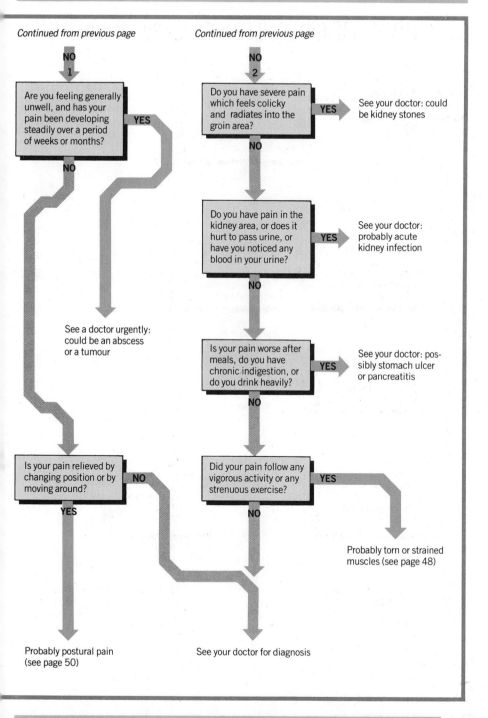

Continued from previous page

NO 1

Are you feeling generally unwell, and has your pain been developing steadily over a period of weeks or months?

YES

See a doctor urgently: could be an abscess or a tumour

NO

Is your pain relieved by changing position or by moving around?

NO

YES

Probably postural pain (see page 50)

Continued from previous page

NO 2

Do you have severe pain which feels colicky and radiates into the groin area?

YES — See your doctor: could be kidney stones

NO

Do you have pain in the kidney area, or does it hurt to pass urine, or have you noticed any blood in your urine?

YES — See your doctor: probably acute kidney infection

NO

Is your pain worse after meals, do you have chronic indigestion, or do you drink heavily?

YES — See your doctor: possibly stomach ulcer or pancreatitis

NO

Did your pain follow any vigorous activity or any strenuous exercise?

YES

Probably torn or strained muscles (see page 48)

NO

See your doctor for diagnosis

NECK, SHOULDER OR ARM PAIN

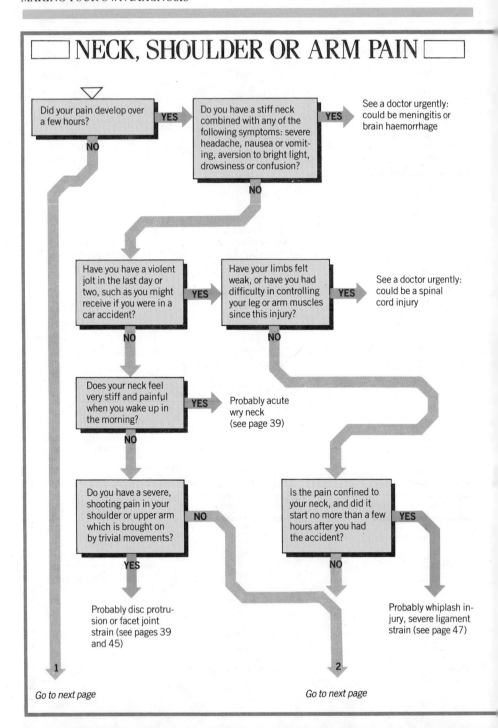

Did your pain develop over a few hours? — **YES** → Do you have a stiff neck combined with any of the following symptoms: severe headache, nausea or vomiting, aversion to bright light, drowsiness or confusion? — **YES** → See a doctor urgently: could be meningitis or brain haemorrhage

NO

NO

Have you have a violent jolt in the last day or two, such as you might receive if you were in a car accident? — **YES** → Have your limbs felt weak, or have you had difficulty in controlling your leg or arm muscles since this injury? — **YES** → See a doctor urgently: could be a spinal cord injury

NO

NO

Does your neck feel very stiff and painful when you wake up in the morning? — **YES** → Probably acute wry neck (see page 39)

NO

Do you have a severe, shooting pain in your shoulder or upper arm which is brought on by trivial movements? — **NO** → Is the pain confined to your neck, and did it start no more than a few hours after you had the accident? — **YES**

YES

NO

Probably disc protrusion or facet joint strain (see pages 39 and 45)

Probably whiplash injury, severe ligament strain (see page 47)

1

Go to next page

2

Go to next page

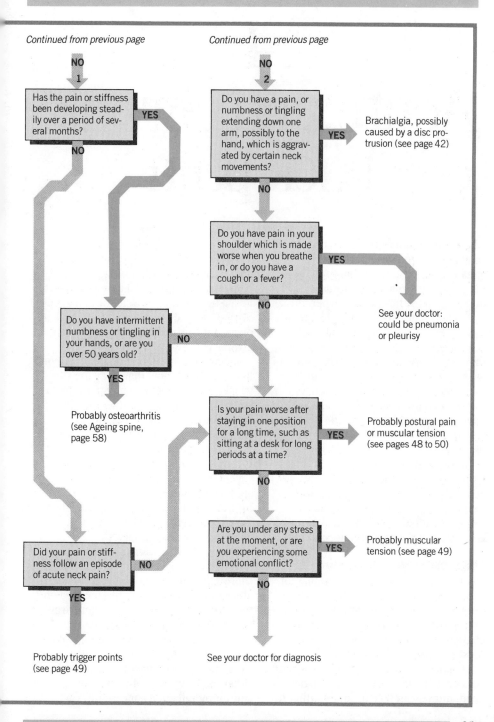

Continued from previous page

NO 1

Has the pain or stiffness been developing steadily over a period of several months? — **YES**

NO

Continued from previous page

NO 2

Do you have a pain, or numbness or tingling extending down one arm, possibly to the hand, which is aggravated by certain neck movements? — **YES** → Brachialgia, possibly caused by a disc protrusion (see page 42)

NO

Do you have pain in your shoulder which is made worse when you breathe in, or do you have a cough or a fever? — **YES**

NO

See your doctor: could be pneumonia or pleurisy

Do you have intermittent numbness or tingling in your hands, or are you over 50 years old? — **NO**

YES

Probably osteoarthritis (see Ageing spine, page 58)

Is your pain worse after staying in one position for a long time, such as sitting at a desk for long periods at a time? — **YES** → Probably postural pain or muscular tension (see pages 48 to 50)

NO

Are you under any stress at the moment, or are you experiencing some emotional conflict? — **YES** → Probably muscular tension (see page 49)

NO

Did your pain or stiffness follow an episode of acute neck pain? — **NO**

YES

Probably trigger points (see page 49)

See your doctor for diagnosis

4
Acute and chronic back pain

There may be no warning whatsoever of an attack of agonizing back pain. Perhaps you stretched just that little bit too high to lift down a heavy suitcase, or you dug the garden for too long when the soil was waterlogged, or your perfect tennis stroke went wrong. Sometimes backache arises from an incident so trivial that you don't really know what you did wrong: was it the way you got out of bed, was it the time you leaned over your armchair to pick up a magazine, or have you been ignoring a little ache for a few days and carrying on with your busy life as usual?

In acute episodes of back trouble the pain generally comes on suddenly and goes, if not quickly enough for your liking, at least within a few days or weeks. Unfortunately, backache can become a chronic or recurring problem.

Diagnosing your back pain

The flow-chart in the previous chapter will have given you a rough idea of the possible cause of your symptoms. It is not meant as a do-it-yourself diagnosis chart: it will simply guide you to the most relevant section in this chapter.

Diagnosing what has gone wrong and which particular part of the back has been injured can be extremely difficult,

even for a specialist. If you have been overdoing things at home or at work and find yourself immobilized with pain, you might have damaged a disc, torn a ligament or muscle, or damaged several of the components of the back at once, but this may not show up on an ordinary X-ray.

Doctors know a great deal more about back problems now than they did fifty years ago, when almost any pain that resulted from an injury to the lower back would be described as "sciatica" or "lumbago", without any clear idea, in most cases, of what had gone wrong. Lumbago simply means sudden and severe pain felt in the lower (lumbar) spine, and nowadays is applied to disc injuries and facet joint strains. Sciatica is a sharp, shooting pain in the leg, caused by a pinched nerve.

The healing process that follows a muscle or ligament injury is now more thoroughly understood, and a considerable amount of research has focused on the disc, its functions and structure and the way in which it ages. Almost all spinal problems are caused by mechanical breakdowns, in other words part of the structure is damaged or out of place. Relatively few cases of back pain are caused by infections or diseases.

DISC PROBLEMS

Although discs are very strong, they are vulnerable to twisting forces, which can rupture the outer layer of cartilage, thus allowing the pulpy gel inside to protrude, hence the term disc protrusion, or disc prolapse. This can cause local pain by irritating the ligaments and the dural sheath, and sometimes the disc presses on a nerve, causing severe pain down an arm or a leg. A disc becomes herniated when part of the nucleus has become completely detached from the main nucleus. Disc problems are most common in the lower back, but they can also occur in the neck or, more rarely, in the middle back.

TYPES OF DISC PROTRUSION

A damaged disc can protrude in several different ways, but it need not be painful. Symptoms depend on the nature of the damage, the amount of nucleus that is protruding and the surface it is pressing against. The outer layers of fibre, the annulus fibrosus, which keep the gel-like nucleus in position, have virtually no pain-sensitive nerves. Therefore, any ruptures in these fibres are probably painless. Only when the nucleus has protruded far enough to press against the ligament, or some other sensitive surface, is it painful. As the disc degenerates with age, small splits frequently occur in the annulus fibrosus, but these are usually painless.

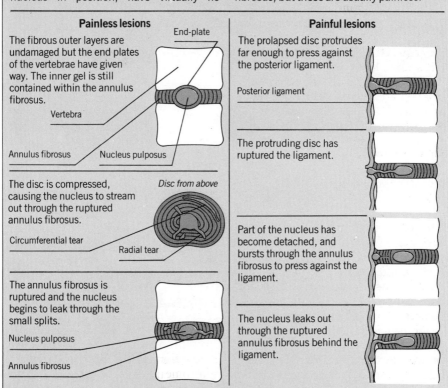

Painless lesions

The fibrous outer layers are undamaged but the end plates of the vertebrae have given way. The inner gel is still contained within the annulus fibrosus.

End-plate

Vertebra

Annulus fibrosus   Nucleus pulposus

The disc is compressed, causing the nucleus to stream out through the ruptured annulus fibrosus.

Disc from above

Circumferential tear

Radial tear

The annulus fibrosus is ruptured and the nucleus begins to leak through the small splits.

Nucleus pulposus

Annulus fibrosus

Painful lesions

The prolapsed disc protrudes far enough to press against the posterior ligament.

Posterior ligament

The protruding disc has ruptured the ligament.

Part of the nucleus has become detached, and bursts through the annulus fibrosus to press against the ligament.

The nucleus leaks out through the ruptured annulus fibrosus behind the ligament.

DISC PROTRUSIONS

This type of injury is popularly known as a "slipped disc", but this term is misleading because it suggests that the disc has slipped out from between the vertebrae, rather like a loose washer. Such movement is impossible, since the disc is bound to the vertebrae by its fibrous outer layers. However, such an injury may cause pain at some distance from the damaged area, and little or no local pain. Medical opinion is divided as to whether this type of acute pain in the lower spine is generally caused by a disc protrusion or by an acute strain or malalignment of one of the facet joints. The term "lumbago" can apply to both disc and facet joint injuries in the lower back.

Disc problems are fairly common, and the more severe protrusions generally affect young and middle-aged adults. This is perhaps because their discs contain a higher proportion of pulpy gel in the centre than those of elderly people, whose discs have dried out. Therefore, if the outer layers of a young person's disc rupture, more gel can be extruded. See page 59 for problems connected with discs in old age.

In the lower back

There may be little or no warning of an acute disc protrusion in the lower back. However, once the damage has been done, you will probably be able to recall that you have recently performed some bending or twisting action, such as pulling up a weed in the garden or moving some furniture, which resulted in either acute pain and an inability to move, or a gradual onset of stiffness, followed after an interval by an acutely painful back.

The pain tends to be of the deep, dull, aching kind, which may be felt in the middle of the lower back or to one side, it may radiate deep into the buttock, hip or groin, and you may have

Causes of disc prolapse
Most painful disc protrusions develop from non-painful ones. An awkward twisting or bending movement compresses the disc first on one side, then suddenly on the other. If the nucleus is already leaking through small tears in the annulus fibrosus, this see-sawing of compressional forces causes the nucleus to burst through the annulus.

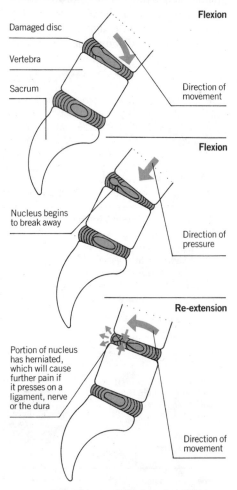

Damaged disc

Vertebra

Sacrum

Flexion

Direction of movement

Flexion

Nucleus begins to break away

Direction of pressure

Re-extension

Portion of nucleus has herniated, which will cause further pain if it presses on a ligament, nerve or the dura

Direction of movement

some aching in your thighs, though these radiating pains may come and go.

You will find certain movements painful and restricted: most people find that it hurts most if they bend forwards, but sometimes bending backwards or to one side may be more painful, and you may find that you lean to one side or are unable to straighten up fully. Quite often, the pain increases suddenly when you cough, laugh, sneeze or strain.

Usually, if you try to walk around, the pain builds up in intensity, particularly if you attempt further bending or reaching movements. Prolonged sitting may offer a temporary relief, but when you try to stand up again the pain and restriction may be even greater. On the other hand though, sitting may be excruciatingly painful, depending on how the disc is protruding. Often, the back pain is continuous but it can be relieved partially or completely by lying flat (though not necessarily on your back).

The disc protrusion may return to its normal position spontaneously in a few days or it may take several weeks. This depends partly on the size and position of the protrusion but also on your own

response to the pain: if your muscles tense up, you will find it increasingly difficult to become mobile again and your recovery will be delayed. If, however, the pain is very severe and you are scarcely able to move, you must lie down and rest your spine: when you are standing the upper part of your body presses down on the disc.

About 50 per cent of sufferers get better within two to four weeks no matter what treatment is given; 90 per cent will have recovered within six weeks. Some of the treatments discussed later in this book may, however, hasten your recovery. These include mobilizing exercises (see page 159), manipulation to reduce pain and improve mobility, and acupuncture, which also helps to reduce pain and to relax muscles. Traction can also be a help in some cases.

A problem to bear in mind is that here – as with so many types of back pain – even the experts cannot agree, and there is a great deal of controversy about how many of the people who suffer from the above set of symptoms actually have a protruding disc. Some would say that it is as few as 5 per cent, while others would go as high as 90 per cent. Similar symptoms can be caused by the facet joints or other problems involving pressure on nerves.

In the mid back
Disc protrusions in this part of the spine are rare because it is less mobile, but they do occur occasionally, in which case they generally require prolonged traction or surgery.

In the neck
In a typical attack of acute neck pain, you will wake up first thing in the morning and find that you are unable to lift your head from the pillow or that it is

POSSIBLE SITES OF PAIN

A disc protrusion usually causes severe pain around the site of injury and a wider area of dull ache that may spread some distance from the injury. Generally the pain is limited to just one side of the body, according to the direction of the protrusion. Here we show pain for the right hand side of the body.

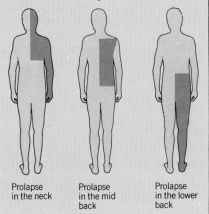

Prolapse in the neck

Prolapse in the mid back

Prolapse in the lower back

extremely painful and difficult to turn your head one way or the other. Usually, it is equally difficult to bend your head backwards or forwards.

The condition is often referred to as wry neck, or torticollis, and the restricted movement is typical of a problem caused by a physical derangement rather than a disease. The term can also apply to facet joint strain (see page 44), and some experts still regard it as a form of muscle spasm.

Normally, you will feel better within five to ten days without any particular treatment, though once again recovery can be hastened by gentle manual traction from a manipulative therapist, by wearing a soft collar at night to prevent further strain, acupuncture to relieve muscle tension and mobilizing exercises, (see Chapters 8, 11 and 14).

Wry neck can occasionally occur in young children, in which case it may be caused by an infection of the throat or ear. Elderly or late middle-aged people rarely suffer from acute wry neck: the symptoms at this age tend to become chronic and are part of the general process of degeneration.

Although wry neck is painful and unpleasant, you should be able to continue work and other normal activities.

CHRONIC DISC PROLAPSE

Occasionally, a prolapsed disc does not return to its original position, but stays bulging out of line, resulting in chronic back trouble if it presses against the sensitive posterior ligament or the lining of the spinal cord, the dural sheath. If the disc has been injured, it cannot heal properly, and fibrous scar tissue may be another cause of chronic back pain and stiffness.

Disc cartilage contains a few pain-sensitive nerves in the outer layers so it is possible that pain can be felt directly from irritation at that source. The pain is much more likely to be produced by irritation of the dura and the adjacent ligaments. These problems typically follow episodes of severe pain caused by a protruding disc.

In the lower back

This problem in the lumbar spine will probably cause aching and stiffness after you have been sitting down. You may also feel sharp twinges, and occasionally your back might "lock" in one position. The pain is usually located on one side of the back and you may also have some intermittent leg pain, possibly with pins and needles in your legs. These symptoms, combined with a background of dull aching, are common in middle-aged back sufferers and may often be provoked by postural strains or excessive lifting and bending.

Your long term outlook is quite good because as you progress into late middle age or old age, the spine will stiffen and the ligaments will ossify, which makes the overall structure much more stable. In the intervening years, however, you will probably want to seek relief from the various therapies that are available, including manipulation, traction and acupuncture. A few people may need surgery. Above all, though, you should do regular exercises to minimize the stress on the spine (see pages 157 to 159), improve your posture and avoid any activities or sports which may put your back at risk.

In the neck

Similar problems can occur in the neck. You may find that after two or three episodes of acute neck pain early in your adult life, as you approach middle age, perhaps becoming less fit and with more work stress and tension in your life, you develop frequent deep aching in the shoulder and upper back area. Every now and again you may experience a milder version of the stiff and painful neck. You might notice grinding and graunching noises on sudden movements of the head and neck. The cause of this is a combination of thinning of the discs, greater compression strain on the small joints at the back of the neck and strained ligaments.

Once the disc thins, the ligaments become slacker and can no longer fulfil their normal stabilizing function, thus making that whole segment of the spine less stable. You may also suffer from intermittent nerve root pain, perhaps with pins and needles in one or both hands, caused by temporary compression of the nerve roots. The treatment for the neck is similar to that for the lower spine, though you are more likely to develop patterns of chronic muscular tension in the neck area and must try to prevent this happening by learning how to relax thoroughly (see the special relaxation techniques on page 171).

COMPRESSED NERVES

Sometimes, when a disc bulges to one side, it presses on one of the nerve roots which exit from the spinal column. If this happens, you will feel pain not only in the immediate area, but also wherever the nerve leads to, usually the leg or arm on that side. A pinched nerve can cause other disturbances of sensation as well, such as numbness or pins and needles. If this goes on for a long time, the nerve root can be permanently damaged, and the muscles controlled by that nerve will become weaker. The sheath containing the nerve can swell as a reaction to being pinched.

Sciatica

If a disc in your lower back is pressing on the sciatic nerve, you will feel pain

Compressed nerve
The nucleus of the disc protrudes between the vertebrae and pinches a nerve as it leaves the spinal canal. Pain can occur along the entire length of the nerve.

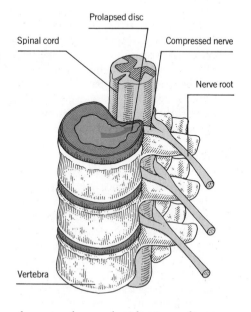

Prolapsed disc

Spinal cord

Compressed nerve

Nerve root

Vertebra

down one leg, and perhaps numbness or tingling in a small area of the leg or foot. In more severe cases when the nerve is damaged, certain muscle groups in the leg may be weakened.

Although this problem usually starts with back pain, after a few days the pain in the back decreases but becomes correspondingly severe in the leg. This indicates that the disc has protruded even further, or has shifted towards the side of the joint.

In some cases of sciatica, the pain is severe and unrelenting, no matter what position you adopt. However, the pain may well subside if you simply rest in bed. Most disc protrusions resolve spontaneously with time and rest. The pulpy centre of the disc withers away, and the fibrous outer layers fit back into place. After a while, the pain in your leg will ease, and the tingling will gradually disappear. You might be left with a small patch of numbness in your foot, and perhaps some residual weakness when pulling up your foot or your big toe.

About 90 per cent of severe cases of sciatica clear up within three months, but if there is no improvement after two weeks' rest in bed, you should consult your doctor. Manipulation, traction, acupuncture, careful posture and exercises can be tried, but are usually not as successful as injections. A tiny minority may eventually need surgery.

Brachialgia

As with sciatica, the pain can be caused by a protruding cervical disc bulging sideways and pressing on a nerve root as it exits from the spinal canal. This will cause severe pain in your arm or hand, according to which nerve is compressed. It may be accompanied by pins and needles or a patch of numbness. If the nerve root is damaged, causing weakness or loss of muscular reflex, your pain may be very severe and will not settle easily with rest, manipulation or acupuncture. In this case you are quite likely to be given a collar to wear, and you may need to rest in bed with your head in continuous traction. Alternatively, you may be given an injection. See page 108 for details on treatment.

CHRONIC SCIATICA AND BRACHIALGIA

Prolonged sciatic pain may be caused by a continuing disc protrusion, epidural root fibrosis, or lateral canal stenosis (see page 59). Chronic brachialgia may be caused in any of these ways, but in very rare cases there may be other explanations. The cervical nerves can be trapped between the collar bone and the first rib, by an extra rib (cervical rib), or by a tumour at the base of the neck.

NERVE PATHWAYS

The sciatic nerves run from the base of the spine to the feet, leaving the spinal canal between the fourth lumbar and second sacral vertebrae. If one of these nerves is pinched, you will feel sharp, shooting pain down one leg, perhaps combined with numbness or pins and needles. The brachialgic nerves leave the spinal canal between various cervical vertebrae, and run from the base of the neck to the hands. Pressure on one of them will cause severe pain down that arm, even to the hand, with numbness or pins and needles. In either case, certain muscles in the affected limb may also become weak.

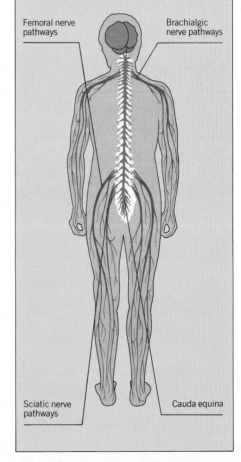

Femoral nerve pathways

Brachialgic nerve pathways

Sciatic nerve pathways

Cauda equina

Continuing disc protrusion

In a small number of cases of sciatica and brachialgia, the disc does not return to its original position, but continues to press on the nerve. If your pain does not subside after six weeks of rest and conservative treatment, you should go to see an orthopaedic surgeon or a neurosurgeon. He may perform a myelogram (see page 78) to find out which of your discs is prolapsed. Depending on the degree of your pain, the extent of nerve damage, and your general disability, he might recommend an operation to remove the protruding part of the disc. Occasionally, a piece of disc cartilage can become completely detached and lie wedged against the nerve. Myelography does not always detect this problem, and further investigations, such as CT scanning (see page 81), may be necessary. Once diagnosed, the fragment can be removed by surgery.

If chronic sciatica is caused by a detached fragment of cartilage, manipulation, traction, acupuncture and rest rarely have any lasting benefit, and even spinal injections, such as epidurals (see page 105), relieve the symptoms at most for just a short while. Your problem is how to cope with chronic sciatic pain. Remaining in severe pain for a long period of time can affect not only your psyche but also your work and your family life. This will be dealt with more fully later (see Chapter 15). Chronic brachialgia is more likely to resolve spontaneously, though it may take six to nine months.

Epidural root fibrosis

When a protruding disc returns to its original position, the nerve root sheath may be scarred from inflammation and bruising, and might become attached to the walls of the spinal canal. If this happens, although the continuous pain

Epidural root fibrosis

Inflexible scar tissue growing on the injured dura can become attached to the bony walls of the spinal canal, trapping the nerve root. This makes any bending movements, which pull on the nerve, very painful.

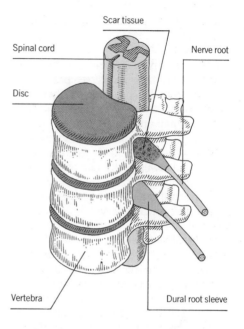

Scar tissue

Spinal cord

Nerve root

Disc

Vertebra

Dural root sleeve

in the limb will diminish, it may return when you bend over. Usually, the pain is relieved simply by straightening up or lying down flat. As the months go by, however, the range of movement does not increase since the scar tissue is firm. In some cases the nerve root will become free in time and your range of motion can then increase. If this does not happen, you may need to undertake a programme of exercises designed to stretch the fibrous tissue little by little. Sometimes the problem is treated by an orthopaedic surgeon using manipulation under anaesthetic in order to stretch out the nerve root by extreme straight-leg-raising movements. It may also respond to injections of cortisone or steroid (see Chapter 9).

JOINT STRAIN AND MALALIGNMENT

If any joint is twisted or jerked, bones may become slightly displaced, causing severe pain as the ligaments and joint capsule are irritated. The medical term for this malalignment is subluxation.

FACET JOINTS

Acute back pain is often caused by one of the small facet joints (see page 19), which link the vertebrae together, being strained or pushed slightly out of alignment. This type of problem can occur at any level of the spine, but, as with disc trouble, it is more likely to affect the neck and lower back. The pain comes directly from irritation of the facet joints, and if the joint capsule swells up it may pinch a nerve.

In the lower back

An awkward twisting or bending movement may cause injury to the ligaments, muscles and capsule of the facet joints. In a middle-aged person, when the discs have started to degenerate and the ligaments might be rather slack, the facet joints tend to slip out of alignment.

The symptoms of this kind of attack are very similar to those caused by a protruding disc in the lower back, since the pain may be very severe and restrict your movements for the first two or three days. Pain may radiate to your buttock, hip, lower abdomen and thighs, as in the case of a disc protrusion, but without the sharp pain down the leg felt when one of the sciatic nerve roots is trapped, and without any numbness or weakness in an arm or leg.

This type of problem responds to rest, pain-killers, exercise and manipulation. As in cases of minor disc protrusion, a great deal depends on your general state of health and fitness. If you have good muscle tone and are able to

FACET JOINT MALALIGNMENT

A joint is malaligned if the bones have slipped slightly out of line but still overlap at some point along the surface of the joint. This differs from dislocation, a condition in which the bones no longer make contact at any point along the surface of the joint.

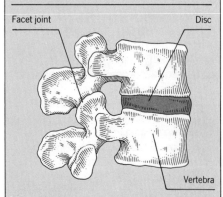

Facet joint   Disc

Vertebra

Normal joint
In a normal facet joint, above, the flat bony surfaces of the articular processes of two vertebrae line up exactly.

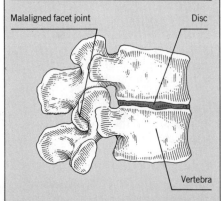

Malaligned facet joint   Disc

Vertebra

Malaligned joint
When the joint is malaligned, above, the bones have slipped slightly, so that the surfaces no longer align properly.

relax properly, you will probably recover more quickly than someone with slack muscles or someone who tenses up in response to pain.

In the mid back

Awkward twisting or bending strains may also set up acute mid-back pain, radiating like a girdle round the side and even to the front of the chest or upper abdomen. Initially, it can be so severe that it is painful even to breathe.

The same set of causes may be involved here as in other spinal problems; for example, a squash player who did not warm up and was over-vigorous in his strokes might develop this type of pain some hours afterwards. If you are moving house and are busy lifting furniture, you are also at risk. Sometimes this problem can develop if you simply turn over in bed at night or sleep awkwardly. Even after the initial pain and restriction have eased, a lot of people feel some residual pain and find that their movements continue to be limited for weeks, months or even years unless they have received adequate treatment, which in this case generally entails manipulation (see Chapter 8).

Mid-back pain of a less severe nature is relatively common and may occur at almost any age, though it more often affects young and middle-aged adults. You will usually feel better if you adopt a suitable position, but will soon be reminded of it when you try to change position or turn in a particular direction. This type of pain is variously caused by the facet joints, minor disc protrusions or rib lesions, when the joints between the ribs and the backs of the thoracic vertebrae are malaligned.

In the neck

Problems involving any of the joints in the neck will make your neck very stiff and painful. This condition has very similar symptoms to a disc protrusion in the neck, and the term "wry neck" can apply to both types of problem. If you have a facet joint strain in the neck, it will be painful and your movements will be limited in certain directions when you turn or bend your head to one side.

Most people find it more comfortable to lie down, taking the weight of the head off the neck, but others find that this makes it even worse. The solution here is to keep the neck supported: try a soft collar, or roll and twist a towel and use it to stop your head lolling from side to side when you sleep (see page 69). This will ease the pain, and facilitate the healing process.

These episodes rarely lead to any long-term problems, but sometimes after weeks or even months pain may persist, together with restricted movement and aching extending into the shoulder-blade area. Trigger point areas may develop (see page 49), but on the whole manipulation is extremely useful in settling this type of case. Although the difference will not show up on an X-ray, it is possible for an experienced manipulator to detect whether the facet joints are just sprained or are actually out of alignment.

SACROILIAC JOINT STRAIN

This most commonly occurs in young to middle-aged women, though men, in particular sportsmen, may also suffer from this problem. The reason why this injury is more common among women is probably related to pregnancy, since the tough fibrous ligament of the sacroiliac joint, which links the spine to the hip, tends to relax during pregnancy, in preparation for childbirth.

The initial cause of a sacroiliac strain may be a twisting or bending movement, and you can also do the damage if

SACROILIAC JOINT

The fused spinal segments which make up the sacrum have two crescent shaped surfaces, one on each side, the articular surfaces of the sacrum. These fit snugly into two corresponding surfaces, one on each hip bone. Together the two hip bones and the sacrum make up the pelvic girdle. The female pelvis is shown here, the male's is slightly narrower and deeper. The thigh bones fit into the sockets on each hip bone.

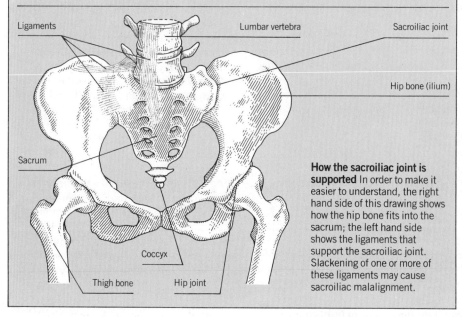

Ligaments

Lumbar vertebra

Sacroiliac joint

Hip bone (ilium)

Sacrum

Coccyx

Thigh bone

Hip joint

How the sacroiliac joint is supported In order to make it easier to understand, the right hand side of this drawing shows how the hip bone fits into the sacrum; the left hand side shows the ligaments that support the sacroiliac joint. Slackening of one or more of these ligaments may cause sacroiliac malalignment.

you step off a kerb unexpectedly, so that your muscles are not prepared for the strain, so the ligaments absorb the force.

Once the sacroiliac joint is strained or dislodged, you will feel a sharp pain in the upper inner area of the buttock when you put your foot down or strike the heel on that side. There will also be a background, wedge-shaped area of pain, radiating deep into the lower buttock. If the pain is severe, it may travel further down the back of the thigh. No major nerves are pinched, so there will be no numbness or weakening of the muscles, and in general this problem does not cause very severe pain. It can, however, be a nagging nuisance that aches even when you are resting.

Many of these acute strains will settle down spontaneously within a week or two, but if they persist they will generally respond quickly to manipulation. However, if the ligament has been strained more than once or twice, there is a likelihood of long-term twinges or aches with occasional flare-ups. There are effective ways of tightening the ligaments with sclerosant injections, in order to hold the joint more firmly.

If the symptoms have been going on for longer than a month, it would be wise to go to your doctor for a check-up in case you have a chronic inflammation rather than just a sprained joint, though you will probably be well aware of when the pain started and what caused it.

LIGAMENT INJURIES

It is unlikely that an attack of back pain would be due entirely to strained ligaments. However, there are certain types of injury in which ligaments may be the main cause of pain. Ligaments do not heal easily, because they have a limited blood supply. They can take longer to heal than a fractured bone. Indeed, they often fail to heal completely, leaving residual scar tissue and adhesions (matted fibrous tissue which prevents the ligaments from gliding over the surface of the bone). This can become a source of chronic pain.

Slack or strained ligaments

In old age, the discs become thinner (see page 59), bringing the vertebrae closer together. The ligaments which used to support the spine firmly will be slacker, so the joints are looser. Ligaments become slack during pregnancy, and an injury to the spine can also dislodge joints. Once this happens, there is a strong likelihood that the facet joints will become dislodged from time to time (see page 44). It is all rather like a worn machine with a loose drive belt or pulley: any undue strain will probably throw something out of gear.

Minor strains and changes of position cause a feeling of the back "going out", or locking, and cause a sharp pain combined with a deep diffused ache. Frequent locking episodes in the neck or lower back are due to instability.

The locking sensation comes from the facet joints being dislodged. If the disc is also involved, prolonged bending or stooping activities will cause pain and stiffness, and you may not be able to straighten up. If you suffer from this condition, your lifestyle is likely to be affected: gardening and do-it-yourself jobs can become a problem.

If your ligaments are also strained or weak, you will feel pain after prolonged sitting and inactivity, and a change of position will tend to spark off acute twinges. Ligaments are weakest at the ends, where they are attached to the bone, and this is where they can be overstretched. They will then become inflamed and cause a background ache much of the time. This pain will probably be most severe first thing in the morning, but wears off when you move around. It is aggravated by vigorous exercise or activity, but also increases if you sit still for a long time.

This type of back pain is difficult to cope with since you never seem to be entirely free of trouble. The response to treatment is variable, but attention to your posture, general fitness and good muscle tone, as well as exercises (see pages 157 to 158), can all help.

Each acute episode can be dealt with in the usual ways (rest, use of a collar or corset, exercises, manipulation or acupuncture – if you are having frequent attacks of pain, you will get to know what works best for you), but lasting effects can be achieved only by stabilizing the unstable segments. Ligament sclerosant therapy (see page 104) comes into its own for this. An alternative is regular home traction on an inversion traction machine. Surgery in the form of spinal fusion (see page 113) is a less common treatment for ligament injuries than it used to be.

As you become older, your spine usually becomes more stable again, because your ligaments will tend to harden, and the whole structure becomes stiffer.

Whiplash syndrome

This happens when the ligaments surrounding joints in the neck are strained or possibly ruptured. It may happen if the head is bent violently backwards or forwards – as might happen in a car accident, for example. The muscles are not poised to absorb the shock, so the joints are forced to the extreme of their range, which is limited by the ligaments. The ligaments thus absorb the impact. Other parts of the neck, such as discs, muscles and vertebrae, can also be damaged in this type of accident.

Many cases of whiplash syndrome pass unnoticed initially, because an X-ray will not reveal damage to ligaments, and internal bleeding may be very slow. However, over a number of hours, perhaps overnight, the neck becomes very stiff and painful.

It is important to start treating this condition in its early stages, because otherwise it can create long-term problems. If there is any likelihood that you have suffered a whiplash injury, consult your doctor, who will probably advise you to rest, prescribe pain-killers, and perhaps give you a collar to wear for a few days. The best form of early treatment is manual traction given by a manipulative therapist.

Cause of whiplash injury
A car accident, in which the car is bumped from behind, can cause the head to be jerked violently backwards and forwards without any warning, resulting in overstretched and/or torn ligaments.

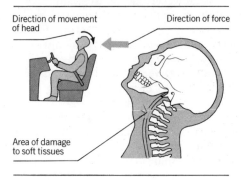

Direction of movement of head

Direction of force

Area of damage to soft tissues

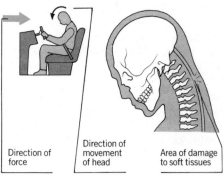

Direction of force

Direction of movement of head

Area of damage to soft tissues

MUSCULAR STRAINS

Injuries to the muscles in the back and neck are not as common as most people imagine. Many painful conditions of the back are often described by doctors as "muscular" or "ligamentous". To some extent this description may be true, since the muscles and ligaments are part and parcel of the workings of the back and can be affected by undue tension and associated strain. Tense muscles may be incidental to a disc protrusion or facet joint strain.

A purely muscular injury to the back typically happens to an athlete under-

taking vigorous exercise after insufficient stretching and warming up. The pain will probably start quite suddenly, and will recur after repetition of the action that initially triggered it. Reaching or pulling movements are likely to aggravate it, and the muscles might be tender and slightly swollen. There may be some internal bleeding if the muscle is injured.

Muscular strains can be a nuisance, but they usually respond to rest and physiotherapy. Few muscular injuries take more than a fortnight to heal.

Chronic muscular tension

Occasionally, muscles become chronically tense. This is usually a result of
poor posture, and is common among
people who spend hours leaning over
a desk, such as typists or computer
operators, and people such as factory
operators who stand or sit for long
periods with their arms outstretched
manipulating small objects.

If your work involves such posture,
it is very important to ensure that your
desk or work surface and your chair are
the right height for you. If you are tall,
you will inevitably have to drop your
head and shoulders a little further to
reach a working height that is designed
for an average-sized person. This may
impose greater strain on the muscles
which are constantly working to support
the load. Tense muscles may be relaxed
through massage or exercises to stretch
them (see Chapter 14).

If you are engaged in a task that
involves constantly repeating the same
pattern of movements in the arms and
shoulders, for instance working on a
production line, the muscles naturally
become tired. When this happens, the
vulnerable trigger point areas (see overleaf) may tighten up and start referring pain to other areas. This is slightly
different from the static postural pain
that a draughtsman can develop poring
over his drawings, but both are tests of
endurance of muscle, one through
repetitive action and the other through
sustained position.

Psychological stress is a factor in
determining which individual performing the same activities in the same place
of work is most susceptible to developing chronic neck pain, shoulder pain or
headaches. A high level of anxiety and
frustration can cause an increase in
muscular tension, particularly in the
neck. If you are unable to release these

tensions, either vocally or through some
physical outlet, you might suppress
your emotions by tensing your muscles.

Most people who develop neck pain
will at some time or other raise the
question "Is it because of the draught I
was in from that open window in the car
or the cold corridor I was standing in for
an hour or two last night?". This is a
common supposition and there is an
element of truth in it: cold draughts or
winds, by rapidly cooling the skin and
superficial muscles, cause an increase in
muscular tension, which reduces the
blood flow. The combination of these
factors can contribute towards the
development of trigger points, which
are described below.

Certain beverages such as coffee,
which stimulates the nervous system,
can cause increased excitability of the
muscles, which in turn makes them
more likely to contract over a period of
time. Excessive alcohol fatigues your
muscles, and over a long period it can
even damage the muscle cells. It has
recently been recognized that, in susceptible people, certain foods can cause
abnormal reactions involving the muscles,
producing widespread muscular aching.
Unless you are aware of this possibility,
it may very well remain an undetected
cause of your back pain.

Trigger points

Pain from spinal structures can radiate to
surrounding areas and set up secondary
points of tension, which become taut
little bands or knots in the muscle. This
used to be called fibrositis but is now
referred to as trigger point phenomena
or, somewhat dauntingly, myofascial
dysfunction. It is very common in the
neck and shoulders of people who are
under postural stress or who are experiencing one of the acute episodes of neck
pain described previously. There are

Trigger points
There are several sites often affected by muscle trigger points. These are some of the most common. The specific trigger points are indicated on the figures as black crosses. The dark red tints are the main areas of referred pain; the lighter tints show the maximum extent of referred pain.

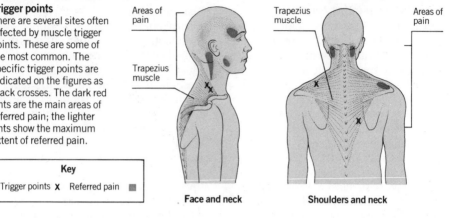

Areas of pain

Trapezius muscle

Trapezius muscle

Areas of pain

Key	
Trigger points **x**	Referred pain ■

Face and neck

Shoulders and neck

recognized common positions at which these trigger points develop, and if you touch one, you will feel a tense, hard nodule which may twitch as a response to deep pressure and spread pain into whichever area of the shoulder, arm or chest is already hurting.

This problem must be approached in several ways. In the first place, if there is any injury to a spinal joint, it must be corrected. If this is not the primary cause, the tender points of the muscle need to be relaxed with massage, physiotherapy or passive stretching exercises, a local injection or acupuncture. Then the circumstances at

work or at home which have caused the problem must be altered to ensure that the tension and pain do not return. This may involve improved seating, or adapting a task so that your back is under less strain. At home, you may have to alter the height of your work surfaces, while in the office it may be necessary for you to obtain stands for books, manuals and documents so that your line of vision is almost horizontal. Ergonomic design – adapting the working environment to suit the person working in it – is an extremely important factor in eliminating back pain due to poor posture. See Chapter 13 for more detailed advice.

POSTURAL PAIN

This is probably one of the most common causes of chronic backache. Pain is the natural result of adopting a position in which one or a group of muscles or ligaments are kept in a state of tension for a sustained period. Postural pain may be caused by prolonged standing, sitting or lying.

If you put your heel on a chair and rest your leg horizontally for 20 to 30 minutes, the chances are that your knee will feel stiff and painful as soon as

you try to move it again. The knee is not designed like a suspension bridge and the ligaments will start to hurt if you stretch them to the limit and expose them to the full force of gravity.

In any mechanical system the weakest points are usually the links or the hinges which allow movement, and just as the hinges of a door will eventually bend or break if the door is constantly slammed, so the ligaments which restrain the joints in your body will start to hurt if you apply unequal, excessive or sustained forces through the joints. Often all that you need to do is to improve your posture and to do exercises aimed at strengthening the muscles used in posture and altering the position of the pelvis (see page 138).

Sway back syndrome

Also known as hollow back, this is a way of standing which often leads to back pain. The abdomen is held forwards, while the bottom is pulled back and upwards, so that the lower back is arched right in. A common factor in this type of case is "hypermobility", or excessive flexibility. Some people have extremely flexible joints, and are liable to suffer from this. Others have let their abdominal muscles slacken with disuse so that the pelvis tilts forward. If they have also been putting on extra weight around the midriff, this will add to the strain. Pregnant women are particularly at risk, and high-heeled shoes, which throw the weight of the body forwards onto the toes, often produce this posture, and thus contribute to backache.

The pain may come from ligaments which are under tension in front of the lower back and from facet joints being pushed together and compressed by the arch that develops in the lower back. You may feel pain in the low back, sometimes radiating round to the lower abdomen and hips and occasionally even to the buttocks and upper thighs. This occurs particularly after standing for a long time. The problem develops gradually and insidiously and you may never experience the sort of acute episode described on page 47, though you may sometimes feel sharp twinges of pain, particularly when you change position, for example, from standing to sitting. The simple cause for this back pain is frequently missed, which is

particularly sad as the cure often lies in improved posture and simple exercises.

Kissing spines

This is another version of the hollow back in which the tips of the spinous processes (the bumps which you can feel down your back) touch and are compressed if the sway-back position is maintained for any length of time.

This tends to cause a more sharply localized pain. Your doctor may be able to discover whether you have this problem by feeling for localized tenderness at the tips of the spinous processes, or he may want to test his diagnosis by injecting a local anaesthetic between the two suspect segments. Improved posture will help, but injections (see page 108) or even surgery may be necessary.

Strains in the neck

This problem can readily occur if you have a sedentary job involving leaning over a desk for long periods with your head bent forward. This puts continuous strain on the muscles of your upper back and neck, probably aggravated by hunched shoulders putting a chronic strain on the trapezius muscle.

This posture would normally strain the muscles rather than the ligaments. It leads to aching in the neck, shoulder and shoulder blade area which develops after some hours and can be relieved by getting up and moving around. After some weeks or months, however, the time comes when moving around no longer relieves the pain and a pattern of chronic muscular tension sets in.

Occasionally, instead of causing neck or shoulder pain, neck strain may give rise to headaches, which develop late in the day or in the evening. This is a typical tension headache, though in this instance produced by physical rather than psychological stress.

VIOLENT INJURY TO THE SPINE

If you fall from a height or are struck by a heavy object anywhere along the length of your spine, there is a risk of major injury to the vertebrae, spinal cord and nerves, which could lead to paralysis or even death since damage to the spinal cord itself means that no neural impulses can be carried below the area of damage. Even if you are able to get up and hobble around, it is still important to consult a doctor who can check that the bones are undamaged by taking an X-ray. Most fractures to the spine, though, are relatively minor; they may not be caused by a particularly violent accident, and you may not even realize that your spine is fractured.

Avulsion

In avulsion, the tip of the transverse or spinous process is cracked or pulled off. This sometimes happens as the result of a violent muscular action: sportsmen are typical victims of this kind of accident. If you have this type of injury, you will feel sudden and severe pain when it first happens, and you should refrain from any activity which provokes the pain until it is healed.

Microfracture

A second type of minor injury is a small fracture, or microfracture, which is a horizontal crack or break through the end-plate of the vertebra or one of the articular processes. It has recently been recognized that even without a violent injury, small fractures can occur, for example, when lifting a heavy weight. Most people do not get the benefit of the special X-ray investigation needed to bring such tiny fractures to light, but if you have a microfracture and are un-aware of it, you may make it worse by taking the wrong treatment: it is not

wise to manipulate or mobilize micro-fractures, since rest is the best treat-ment. The majority of microfractures heal spontaneously, without treatment but people with continuing back trouble may have a microfracture that has failed to unite properly.

Stress fractures

These can occur in the lower back if you are imposing a lot of stress on the spine, for example, through vigorous physical training or athletics – hurdling, pole vaulting or long distance running are typical examples. Microfractures, and occasionally crush fractures, can also be caused in this way. There may be some advance warning in the form of pain or stiffness due to over-use, but when the fracture happens you will probably feel a much more sudden and sharp pain superimposed on the background ache. You will feel a sharp and more severe pain if you repeat the activity that first caused the injury, so you should avoid strenuous activity for six to eight weeks, until the fracture is healed.

Crush fractures

Sometimes a vertebra collapses entirely. This may occur as a result of a violent injury, but a common sufferer is the elderly person who has considerable thinning of the bones (see osteoporosis, page 58), so that the weight of the body itself can cause a vertebra to crumble. If you are elderly and have developed a sudden severe and immobilizing back pain (usually in the mid or lower back) without any particular external injury, then a crush fracture is a possible cause. If you are in severe pain, you should see a doctor. If he suspects a crush fracture, he will probably arrange for you to have an X-ray. After a crush fracture the vertebra becomes wedge-shaped, and this shows up clearly on an X-ray. You may develop an angle or bump in the area of the pain, which will be visible externally, because the bone has wedged in this shape. You will also tend to be bent forwards and the pain may radiate around both sides of your chest or your abdomen.

Initially, the only treatment for this is a combination of pain-killers and rest, but later on there may be a case for instituting some drug therapy (see page 103) to encourage the bone to remineralize. However, once the wedge compression has formed, the resulting hunch is likely to remain. The best way of tackling osteoporosis is to prevent it altogether: stay active into old age for as long as possible, since this encourages the continued renewal of the stronger components of the bone structure.

Coccydinia

A fall onto the coccyx or tail-bone can cause a persistent painful bruising which prevents you from sitting comfortably. Normally, this will heal on its own, but if the pain remains severe after several months, you may need a local injection to reduce inflammation. A tiny minority need surgery.

MINOR FRACTURES

Violent injury to the spine may result in the fracture of a vertebra and consequent damage to the spinal cord. However, many less serious fractures are caused by quite a trivial movement. Minor fractures, which are unlikely to involve damage to the spinal cord but can cause problems nevertheless, fall into three main categories.

Avulsion
One of the processes may be cracked, or the tip can be torn off. This injury is usually caused by continued over-use of the muscle attached to the process, and is almost always confined to the lower back.

Microfracture
The flat end-plate of the vertebra, where it joins the disc, can crack, or a small piece may be broken off one of the articular processes. This is typically caused by combined flexion and rotation forces.

Crush fracture
The body of a vertebra can crumble suddenly. Usually, the front collapses further than the back, so that the vertebra is wedge-shaped, making the spine appear humped.

Vertebra

Fragment of transverse process pulled away by muscle

Muscle

Front view

End-plate fracture

Fractured articular process

Side view

Vertebra collapsed on one side

Spinous process causing bump visible on back

Side view

SPONDYLOLISTHESIS/SPONDYLOLYSIS

Vertebrae in the lower back occasionally slip out of line significantly, and this can cause back pain if the joints or ligaments are irritated. Nerves may become trapped producing leg pain, numbness or pins and needles in the legs.

Spondylolysis

This is a small crack across the neural arch. In some cases the condition is congenital, though even when it is, the abnormality does not become apparent until the child is about six. There may be a hereditary factor – members of a family in which it is present are roughly 25 per cent more likely to suffer from serious spinal disorders. Spondylolysis can also occur as a result of an injury, usually through several falls on to the backside, or through over-use, typically in long-distance runners (see Stress fracture, page 52). As a result of this crack, spondylolisthesis may develop, a condition in which part of the vertebra breaks and slips out of position, forwards or backwards.

SPONDYLOLYSIS AND SPONDYLOLISTHESIS

Initially, spondylolysis is just a minor crack across the narrow bridge of bone between the spinous and inferior articular processes and the transverse and superior articular processes. In spondylolisthesis, this widens to a break, allowing the vertebra to slip out of line. The illustrations below and right show the difference between the two conditions. When it slips, the vertebra may press against a nerve, causing pain along the path of the nerve. Spondylolysis is extraordinarily common among Eskimos: this may be due to an inherited trait or to repeated falls onto ice.

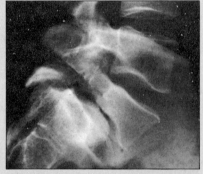

Spondylolisthesis
The X-ray above shows spondylolisthesis in the lumbar spine. Note how the lowest vertebra has slipped out of line.

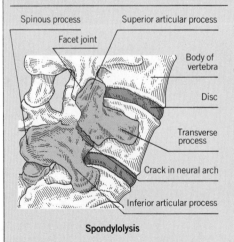

Spinous process — Superior articular process
Facet joint
Body of vertebra
Disc
Transverse process
Crack in neural arch
Inferior articular process

Spondylolysis

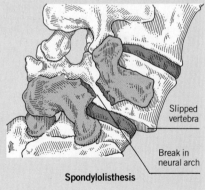

Slipped vertebra
Break in neural arch

Spondylolisthesis

Spondylolisthesis

This is a more severe condition in which the neural arch breaks right through and the vertebra shifts out of place, usually forwards. It is probable that most cases develop from spondylolysis; the crack becomes a break as a result of excessive stresses and strains. Sometimes the vertebra slips gradually as the facet joints wear with age. This condition is called degenerative spondylolisthesis, and it generally affects people aged 50 or over. It develops more frequently in women than in men, and is more common in black people than in whites.

The amount of displacement can be very slight, and there may be no pain whatsoever. However, if a shift in a vertebra is discovered in a growing child, the amount of slippage must be monitored very carefully with an X-ray every six months or so, to detect any further movement. This is important because, if the slip becomes severe while the child is still growing, he may develop an abnormal shape resulting from shortening of the lower back. This generally happens only if one vertebra has moved more than a quarter or half its width. The bones move most rapidly between the ages of ten and 15. Once adolescents have stopped growing, the vertebrae are most unlikely to slip any further. Young people with spondylolysis should avoid contact sports, such as rugby and American football, high diving, and other activities such as judo, with a high risk of back injury. They should also prepare for a career which does not entail lifting.

Both conditions may be treated with a fusion operation (see page 113); in less severe cases a decompression operation (see page 112) is usually successful. In older people, ligament sclerosant therapy (see page 104) helps by tightening ligaments to prevent further slipping. Some people have found that inversion traction (see page 86) is beneficial for minor amounts of displacement.

STRUCTURAL DEFECTS

Some back problems are caused by abnormalities in the structure of the spine. These may be apparent at birth, but many are noticeable only as a child grows. Some are so mild that they cause no symptoms whatsoever, and might never come to light unless the back is examined for some condition unrelated to the structural defect.

Scoliosis

This simply means a sideways curve of the spine, most commonly caused by legs of unequal length, resulting in the pelvis tilting to one side. As a result, the spine compensates by bending slightly towards the higher side in order to bring the level of the shoulders and the head back to horizontal. In fact, as much as 10 per cent of the population have a difference in leg length of a centimetre or more, and although this causes a pelvic tilt and mild compensating curve of the spine, it is unlikely to cause problems, except perhaps in sportsmen such as long distance runners whose spines are frequently being jarred.

If you suffer from sciatica or an acute disc protrusion in the lower back, you may try to minimize the pressure of the bulging disc by bending sideways. This is known as "sciatic scoliosis" and is only a temporary phenomenon which disappears when the disc regains its normal position. However, if you have been suffering from the problem for some time, the muscles and ligaments may become shortened and stiff. This can be treated with manipulation and corrective exercises (see Chapters 8 and 14).

True structural scoliosis is a deformity that arises either in infancy, in which case it can be very severe, or during early adolescence. Vertebrae become narrower on one side, making the spine lean over towards that side and rotate. Much research has been done into the causes but still little is known. It appears to be due to a defect in the growth of the soft tissues supporting the spine. It is important to identify this early on since spinal braces and supports can be worn

---

POSTURAL DEFORMITIES

Abnormalities in the structure of the bones can result in deformed posture. If the vertebrae are narrow on one side, the spine leans over to that side, and in many cases it twists back again a little higher up. This condition is called scoliosis. Vertebrae which are narrow at the front make the spine hunch forwards, a defect which is known as adolescent osteochondritis, or Scheuermann's disease.

Scoliosis
The X-ray on the right shows a spine severely deformed by scoliosis. Milder scoliosis may be apparent only when the person bends forwards, and one shoulder is held higher than the other.

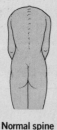 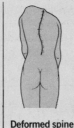

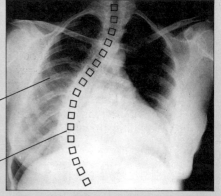

Ribs

Spinal curvature

Normal spine | **Deformed spine**

Scheuermann's disease
The uneven, roughened edges of the vertebrae in the X-ray on the right make the thoracic vertebrae slightly wedge-shaped. This makes the mid back become very rounded and results in a hump-backed appearance.

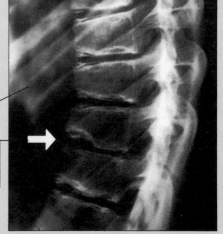

Ribs

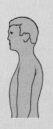 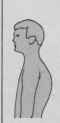

Roughened end-plates

Normal spine | **Deformed spine**

during the growing phase to prevent excessive deformity. If your child's back seems crooked (look at the bare back, with the child standing straight and then bending forwards), or one shoulder blade is more prominent, consult your doctor or the school medical inspector. Occasionally, the deformity is severe enough to require surgical treatment (see page 115).

Mild scoliosis may produce no pain or discomfort initially, but later in life, the accumulation of the unequal stresses and strains may produce a general ache in any part of the back, shoulders or neck and chronic muscular tension patterns can set in. Joints between the vertebrae will degenerate earlier than usual. Most people who have a structural deformity of this kind, however, go through life with no greater incidence of backache than their counterparts with a straight spine.

Adolescent osteochondritis

This is also called Scheuermann's disease, and causes an excessively round-shouldered appearance, or hump-back profile. It tends to occur in adolescents and although the term implies inflammation there is no evidence that it is an inflammatory condition. It frequently develops without any accompanying backache. However, if you or your child become concerned about the deformity, an X-ray will be taken. If osteochondritis is present, it will show up on the X-ray as mottled and roughened areas around the upper and lower surfaces of the vertebrae, usually in the mid spine. There is no truly effective treatment other than corrective postural exercises. The reassuring fact is that the abnormal curvature will stop when the skeleton stops growing, because the disturbance occurs in the parts of the vertebrae that are concerned with bone growth. It is

rare for the deformity to become severe enough to require any kind of spinal corsetry or surgery.

Spina bifida occulta

This is a type of congenital defect which is usually only found if an X-ray is performed for some other reason. There is an absence of bone growth in the neural arch (see page 19), and although some people believe that this is a cause of a "weak back", there is absolutely no evidence for this. It is almost certain that no symptoms of either pain or weakness can ever be attributed to it.

Spina bifida occulta is an innocuous version of the more serious spina bifida, when the spinal cord is exposed or protected only by a thin membrane. This severe condition is always identified at birth or even during pregnancy through ante-natal screening.

Congenital defects

There are some other congenital defects of the spine which need to be mentioned at this point, though again they would be unlikely to be spotted at birth and would come to light only if your back was X-rayed for some other reason. In the first chapter I described the spinal structure which includes five lumbar vertebrae and the five sacral segments which are fused. In some people, the lowest lumbar vertebra is fused with the first sacral segment, resulting in only four motion segments belonging to the lumbar spine. Alternatively, one side of the lowest lumbar vertebra can fuse or form a "false joint" with one side of the first sacral vertebra. The reverse can also occur: the first sacral segment may sometimes becomes isolated from the remaining segments so that it functions as a sixth lumbar vertebra. Generally, these abnormalities cause no problems or symptoms whatsoever.

THE AGEING SPINE

As the spine grows older a number of changes take place, which are given the name osteoarthritis or spondylosis. These are both general terms describing a variety of symptoms; osteoarthritis is completely unrelated to rheumatoid arthritis described on page 64. The main degenerative processes affect the bones and the discs. Bones usually become thinner and more porous, and bony spurs, called osteophytes, often grow on the vertebrae. In a few elderly people, bones thicken irregularly (see Paget's disease, opposite). Discs grow drier and thinner, and ligaments are slacker and less flexible (see Slack ligaments, page 47).

This process is visible under X-ray in about 75 per cent of the population over 50, and usually affects the lower neck and the lower part of the lumbar spine first. Although it is rarely a direct cause of backache, it can give rise to other conditions, described below.

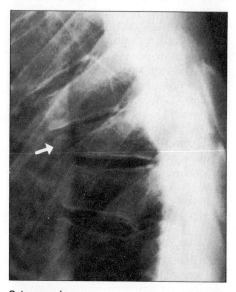

Osteoporosis
The wedge shape of the crushed vertebra is typical of a crush fracture caused by osteoporosis.

Osteoporosis

This has already been mentioned in relation to the development of a crush fracture (see page 52) of the vertebrae, causing an acute episode of back pain. The term simply means thinning out of the bones due to loss of the calcium and mineral structure. It is a gradual process that occurs almost invariably with ageing and tends to accelerate with disuse and immobility. The process of demineralization tends to accelerate after the menopause in women, or following long term use of cortisone and steroids.

Osteoporosis causes problems particularly in elderly people who are immobile, and the best approach is that of prevention: it has been well established that physically active people are far less likely to be affected by osteoporosis,

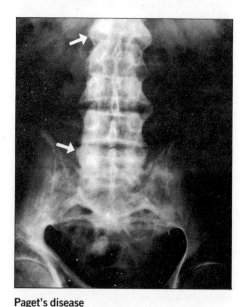

Paget's disease
The denser areas of bone show up white on this X-ray of Paget's disease affecting the lumbar spine.

and therefore you should remain as active as possible throughout your later years. There are some hormone drugs which are advocated to reduce this loss of bone substance, but these are used only in the most severe cases because of the risk of side-effects. Bone salt and mineral replacement drugs, including vitamin D, can be beneficial.

Paget's disease

This is a rare bone disease that tends to occur in the elderly and results in irregular thickening of the outer layer of bone. In this case the reverse of osteoporosis occurs and there is a much greater bone density in these areas. It tends to affect the whole skeleton, though it is possible that the process could start in the spine. However, the first symptoms may well be a pain in the hip, thigh or arm, since Paget's disease is by no means confined to the vertebrae. If this disease is suspected, your doctor will arrange for an X-ray to be taken and this should show the irregular increases in bone density.

Osteophytes

Bony spurs, known as osteophytes, commonly grow on the vertebrae, and sometimes make the central or lateral spinal canal much narrower. This can result in pinched nerves, a condition known as stenosis of the spinal canal. Stenosis of the central canal can be very serious; see page 61 for details.

Lateral canal stenosis may cause sciatica or brachialgia (see page 41), depending on which nerve is pinched. It may not cause constant pain: you will probably feel pain only when you bend backwards or twist your spine, since these movements make the canal even narrower. You will experience intermittent pain down the leg, perhaps with other disturbed sensations including pins and needles or numbness.

Lateral canal stenosis
Bony spurs (osteophytes) form a protruding rim around the edge of the vertebra and the facet joints. They may encroach on the lateral canal, causing stenosis, and can result in a pinched nerve.

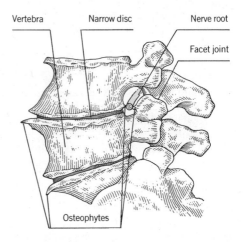

Improved stability may help, and therefore you may benefit from consulting your doctor or a physiotherapist to get advice on posture and exercises to tighten your muscles. More severe cases may need ligament sclerosant therapy (see page 104) to restrict movement of the unstable segments. Very occasionally, surgery is the only answer: the parts of the bone that are narrowing the canal can be removed in a decompression operation (see page 112).

Lateral canal stenosis may also be caused or complicated by a protruding disc which gives a more constant pain (see Compressed nerves, page 41).

Disc degeneration

The fibrous outside of the disc steadily becomes weaker and stiffer with age, while the inside gradually dries out. Until about the age of 50, the nucleus of the disc is still fairly mobile and is liable to prolapse. Beyond about the age of 30, the outer fibres can become weakened allowing the inner pulp to bulge out.

PHASES OF DISC DEGENERATION

Discs are composed mostly of water, but they dry out with age. The process of desiccation is hardly noticeable until around the age of 30, when the outer fibres begin to degenerate and crack. The pulpy nucleus dries out gradually, resulting in much thinner discs by the age of about 60. Although disc protrusions are unusual by this age, thin discs can cause problems, particularly for the facet joints.

Stage 1 (20-30 years)
The nucleus is still healthy, with little loss of fluid content.

Stage 2 (30-40 years)
Outer fibres stiffer, with cracks developing in the outer ring. Fluid content of the nucleus constantly decreasing.

Stage 3 (40-50 years)
Progressive loss of fluid from the nucleus. Outer layers of fibre may have torn.

Stage 4 (50-60 years)
Disc thinner and drier with a very much smaller nucleus; outer fibres stiff and inelastic.

FACET JOINT DISEASE

One result of thinner discs is that the facet joints are jammed closer together and are therefore under much greater pressure. The joints themselves can become irritated and inflamed, and the capsule of lubricating fluid which surrounds each joint might swell and press on a nerve root.

In the lower back

In its early stages, facet joint disease can cause pain in your lower spine when you stand for long periods at a time, and sharp twinges as you change position. You may be unable to adopt certain positions, such as lying on your front. When it is more advanced, you might suffer from continuous backache with acute phases. The symptoms may well be worse in cold weather.

In the early stages, improving your posture and doing appropriate exercises (see pages 157 to 160) can help, but you may need ligament sclerosant therapy (see page 104). Physiotherapy or acupuncture may help. Acute episodes can be treated with manipulation or traction just as for acute disc trouble (see pages 85 and 94). A spinal corset may be helpful. Inflammation of the facet joints can be relieved through injections, and nerves can be deadened by freeze injury techniques (see Facet joint injections, page 108). Operations such as the removal of the facet joints, lateral decompression or spinal fusion (see pages 112 to 113) may help a trapped nerve root.

In the mid back
Acute attacks of pain in the mid back may become chronic unless they are properly treated. If one or two segments become unstable, or the small joints become hyper-irritable, recurrent attacks sometimes become a problem, in which case ligament sclerosant therapy (see page 104) may hold the answer.

In the neck
Similar problems can occur in the neck. In addition to aching accompanied by sharp twinges, you might have pins and needles or numbness in your hands, and sometimes patterns of chronic muscular tension develop. Other symptoms may include disturbed balance, ringing in the ears, headaches, pain referred to the face, side of the neck and ear. If you are over 60, the circulation to your brain can be affected, which causes giddy spells and even blackouts brought on by certain neck and arm movements. This is due to narrowing and compression of the artery to the brain which travels within part of the spinal column.

In the elderly it seems that the stabilization process that takes place in the rest of the spine does not impart such beneficial effects in the neck. You will probably be given a collar to support your neck. Careful posture, exercises, gentle traction, massage and acupuncture may all provide some relief, but are unlikely to cure the condition.

Surgery to the cervical spine is much more risky than in the lower back and therefore it is undertaken less often.

CENTRAL CANAL STENOSIS

The spinal canal containing the nerves sometimes become too narrow. This can result in compressed nerves in the lower spine. It is not so common in the neck since the canal is wider at the top.

Prolapsed disc
Sometimes the bulk of the pulpy central portion of the disc may be forced out into the spinal canal. (This is most common in younger people, because the nucleus of the disc tends to shrink and desiccate with age, so that it is gradually under less pressure.) A protrusion of this kind in the lower back can cause symptoms of chronic sciatica, including pain in the legs accompanied by numbness or weakness. If this is the case, you may need urgent treatment, perhaps surgery, and you should see a doctor as soon as possible.

Degenerative changes
In middle-aged or elderly people, bony outgrowths, called osteophytes, may appear on the vertebrae or facet joints, and discs become thinner. These bony spurs may grow into the spinal canal, which makes the canal much narrower, and can affect blood circulation to the nerves. If this happens, you will feel pins and needles, numbness and heaviness or pain in both legs when you walk or run. These symptoms are relieved by bending forwards, sitting or crouching, because the spinal canal is widened in

these positions. Bending backwards or twisting make the canal even narrower and will cause sharp pain.

Occasionally a decompression operation (see page 112) is necessary to remove the parts of bone which are narrowing the canal.

Congenital trait

Some people are born with a narrower spinal canal than others and therefore are more at risk of nerve compression. The spinal canal can also range from oval to triangular or trefoil in shape.

The triangular and trefoil types allow less room for the spinal nerves.

Those with narrow spinal canals are more at risk of developing chronic back problems or sciatica if a disc ruptures or herniates (see page 37). In this instance what may be a minor episode of back pain or sciatica for one person can be severe or chronic if you have an exceptionally narrow spinal canal. This can afflict young adults as frequently as the middle-aged and elderly. In particularly severe cases, decompression surgery may be necessary (see page 112).

CAUSES OF CENTRAL CANAL STENOSIS

The spinal cord, which runs through the central canal, is extremely sensitive to pressure. Even a small reduction in the diameter of the canal can result in severe pain and other symptoms. It may be narrowed by a protruding disc or osteophytes growing into the space. The canal varies in size and shape along its entire length, it is widest in the neck, before many nerves have branched out. Some people have congenitally narrowed canals, or triangular or trefoil-shaped spaces, which do not leave enough room for the spinal cord and can cause severe pain.

Normal spinal canal
The unobstructed canal allows enough space for the spinal cord .

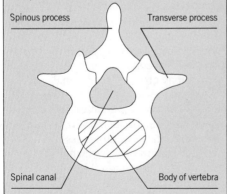

Spinous process

Transverse process

Spinal canal

Body of vertebra

Disc prolapse
The protruding nucleus of a disc encroaches on the central canal.

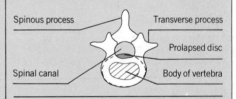

Spinous process

Transverse process

Prolapsed disc

Spinal canal

Body of vertebra

Osteophytes
Bony spurs on the vertebrae grow into the canal resulting in narrowing of the canal.

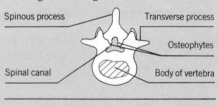

Spinous process

Transverse process

Osteophytes

Spinal canal

Body of vertebra

Congenitally narrow canal
The shape of the vertebrae at birth determines the diameter of the canal.

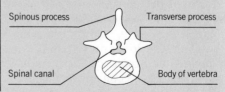

Spinous process

Transverse process

Spinal canal

Body of vertebra

INFLAMMATION AND DISEASE

Diseases and infections account for only a very small percentage of back problems, so if you are otherwise healthy and fit it is extremely unlikely that your backache is caused by any of the following conditions:

● A tumour or cancer can invade the spine or develop in it, as it can in any other organ.

● Sometimes bacterial infection can set up an abscess in or around a vertebra or disc, causing chronic backache.

● Inflammation in the vertebral joints, usually in the neck in rheumatoid arthritis (see page 64) or the sacroiliac joint at the base of the spine, can cause a persisting ache. This usually develops slowly and continues over a long time. It is generally accompanied by increasing stiffness, and it tends not to be relieved by lying down.

If you are unfortunate enough to be one of the tiny minority of those whose back pain is caused by chronic bone infection, a tumour or a serious bone disease, you may get some help from the sections of this book which deal with chronic pain relief, understanding pain, and the emotional aspects of back pain. You should not attempt any treatment without your doctor's advice.

Ankylosing spondylitis

This condition tends to occur in young adults. Joints become inflamed and ligaments calcify to lock the joints rigid. Very little is known about the cause of this condition, but the disease usually affects the sacroiliac joint first, and advances gradually over several years. Eventually the inflammation affects the joints between the ribs and the mid-spine, which reduces chest expansion and makes breathing difficult. However, it is often several years before any

changes show up on X-ray, because progress is very slow.

The first symptoms are pain and stiffness in the lower back and are generally worst first thing in the morning. The pain is usually relieved by moderate exercise (see page 164). You may find it difficult to bend forwards and your hip joints will be stiff.

Your doctor will prescribe some anti-inflammatory drugs and refer you to a physiotherapist for specific exercises to maintain your mobility. You may also benefit from acupuncture. It is very important that this condition is identified early so that your posture and mobility do not deteriorate. It has recently been recognized that this condition occurs almost as often in women as in men, but to a milder degree.

Ankylosing spondylitis
This disease causes the discs and ligaments of the spine to harden gradually and become bone-like; making the spine stiff and inflexible. This extreme stiffness results in a person being hunched forwards with a flat chest and a rounded spine.

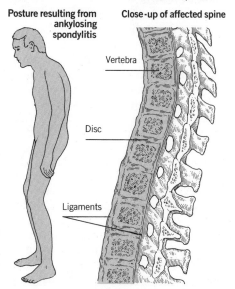

Posture resulting from ankylosing spondylitis

Close-up of affected spine

Vertebra

Disc

Ligaments

Rheumatoid arthritis

This requires a mention at this stage though it is not primarily a disease of the spine and is therefore not discussed elsewhere in this book. It is a general inflammatory arthritis which starts in the small joints of the hands and feet and progresses until it affects the larger joints, such as knees, hips, elbows and shoulders. It does not usually attack the spine until later in its course, and then it usually affects the neck, but by the time it reaches the spine, the diagnosis should already have been made.

It is unlikely that your doctor could mistake this disease for any other spinal disorder, because it will be affecting many other joints before it reaches the spine. If your doctor mentions arthritis when discussing your back, however, he is probably referring not to this but to the normal signs of wear and tear associated with ageing (see page 58), which are not connected with inflammatory arthritis, and therefore will not result in rheumatic disability.

Arachnoiditis

This is an inflammation of the inner lining or dural sheath within the spinal canal, which is usually caused by the introduction of a chemical. It is a rather rare complication of investigations and surgery for the treatment of disc protrusions, which occurred in the past as a result of the use of an oil-based dye in myelographic investigations (see page 78). This dye is no longer used.

It can also be caused by the introduction into the dural sheath of certain antibiotics, crystalloid steroid solutions, and local anaesthetics. However, none of these medications are now used in the general treatment of spinal conditions. A mild infection, or an inflammation caused by bleeding near the exposed dural sheath, may sometimes cause arachnoiditis after a discectomy operation (see page 111).

If you are unfortunate enough to have developed this complication, the symptoms are rather non-specific. They include generalized inflammatory pain, unrelated to movement or posture, and various bizarre sensory disturbances, such as feelings of extreme cold or heat or tingling in the limbs. If you develop any of these symptoms after undergoing investigations or surgery on a disc, you must inform your doctor or specialist immediately. The diagnosis is made by myelography, and you will be given adequate pain-killers until your inflammation subsides.

Infection

This is a rare cause of backache these days. The pain and aching usually develop insidiously over a period of months and are not relieved by lying down or resting. If a large abscess develops in or around the bone or disc, the area is often extremely tender and local muscle might go into spasm at the slightest touch. By the time the infection reaches this severity, there would be some signs of systemic illness, such as fever or general malaise.

Brucellosis, contracted by drinking unpasteurized cows' milk, and tuberculosis are the most common types of infection. Occasionally, there may be an infection within the disc itself, which is called "discitis", and some people suffer from a temporary "discitis", after the use of chymopapain to treat disc prolapse (see page 108). This produces a deep, severe backache, which is exquisitely painful on any movement.

The treatment for an infection in or around the spine is a specific antibiotic taken by mouth or injected directly into the muscles over several weeks to eradicate the infecting organism.

NON-SPINAL CAUSES OF BACK PAIN

Just as problems of the spine can refer pain to other parts of the body, disorders of certain organs may cause back pain. In most cases, these disorders produce other symptoms as well, which make it obvious that the pain does not originate in the spine. One of the characteristics of spinal problems is that the pain is affected by movement and changing position. If your back pain does not alter when you move, the chances are that it is caused by one of the disorders described below.

Influenza and other fevers

Flu normally starts with a feeling of general malaise, mild fever, widespread aches and pains. Fever and headache usually predominate, making the diagnosis obvious. The virus may also cause a sore throat, cough and running nose or indigestion, nausea and diarrhoea. If you have flu, you should rest in bed for a few days. If your fever is very high, causing delirium, rigors and stiff neck, consult your doctor.

Pneumonia and pleurisy

Pain around the lower ribs and towards the back may be the first symptom of a lung infection. Pain may be referred to the tip of your shoulder. You may develop a cough, pain when you breathe in and fever. If you have these symptoms, you should consult your doctor as soon as possible.

Heart attack

This causes severe chest pain which may spread up to the jaw, or down one arm. The pain may also be felt in the back, though it would never be confined to the back. The pain is very severe and is accompanied by any or all of the following symptoms: shortness of breath, nausea, dizziness, feeling faint, feeling cold and palpitations. You need urgent medical attention if you experience these symptoms.

Stomach ulcer

A stomach ulcer may cause a severe burning pain in the mid back, usually worse after fatty or spicy meals. If you have this type of pain, particularly if you also get indigestion, you should consult your doctor.

Inflammation of the pancreas

Excess alcohol can cause inflammation of the pancreas. It produces an intermittent gnawing pain in the mid back, perhaps related to alcohol intake. An alcoholic binge can result in acute inflammation, which causes very severe back or abdominal pain and needs urgent medical attention.

Gall-bladder problems

Gall-stones or inflammation of the gall-bladder can cause pain just below one shoulder blade, usually accompanied by colicky pain in the abdomen, and sometimes nausea and vomiting as well. You may feel referred pain in your right shoulder, perhaps accompanied by fever and shaking. You should consult your doctor if you have any of these symptoms.

Kidney problems

Kidney stones cause intermittent colicky pain in the lower back and nausea. A blockage in the tube from the kidney to the bladder causes pain to the groin or crotch area. If your pain is constant and severe, you have a fever, and your urine is smelly or contains some blood, you probably have a kidney infection. In either case, you should drink plenty of fluids and contact your doctor promptly.

Gynaecological problems

Disorders of the female reproductive organs can refer pain to the low back. Menstrual pain, uterine cramps and pre-menstrual tension can cause a dull, diffuse low back pain. A prolapsed womb produces a dull, dragging ache in the lower back. Infection in the uterus or pelvic tubes may result in backache, abdominal pain, vaginal discharge and pain during intercourse. Most of these disorders cause many other symptoms as well; if your symptoms are severe, you should contact your doctor.

5

Coping with an acute attack

During an acute attack of back pain, there are many ways in which you can help yourself on the road to recovery, whether the attack is caused by a disc or facet joint problem or some other mechanical disorder. Unless this is your first attack, it may not be absolutely essential to see your doctor. Indeed, if you are prone to recurrent back pain, you will probably know what your doctor would advise, so you may not gain very much from seeing him each time.

Time and rest are the essential healers for recovery from an acute attack. As soon as the worst pain has passed, you may be able to begin doing some gentle exercise. Before you start any exercises, however, you must be sure that you are dealing with a simple physical strain or dislodgement. These mechanical disorders tend to run a limited course, unlike some degenerative diseases. This does not mean that you will not benefit from therapies such as exercise, manipulation or traction, all of which are described later; these can be of great value, even when, in some cases, they are just accelerating your inevitable recovery.

WHEN TO CONSULT YOUR DOCTOR

If this is your first ever attack of back pain, it is wise to consult your doctor. However, it is not an emergency that requires him to attend in the middle of the night and you should not expect an instant cure or immediate relief.

Your doctor will want to know about the onset and nature of your pain, its severity, how disabled you are by it, and all the surrounding circumstances. His first task will be to diagnose the cause of your pain, and to discover whether your attack is caused by a mechanical breakdown of some kind, or to a disease. The following chapter, see pages 74 to 81 outlines the doctor's initial examination and describes any other tests which he might perform in order to diagnose your problem. For example, if your pain developed after vigorous exercise you may need to be X-rayed to check whether your bones have been injured.

Urgent cases
The following instances indicate that you should seek medical attention as soon as possible.
● **Unrelenting pain** If you have been

suffering back pain which is not particularly made better or worse by any one movement or position (in other words changes in the stress on the spine), and which is increasing steadily over weeks and months, troubling you day and night, go to see your doctor.

● **Deteriorating muscles** Any profound weakness or wasting away of some of the muscles in either one or both legs (as opposed to a temporary inability to move because of the pain) means that you must see your doctor. This implies considerable nerve damage and it may be accompanied by a weak bladder, incontinence or loss of the sensation of the normal reflex to urinate. The bowel may also be affected in a similar way.

● **General ailing health** If you have been feeling unwell for some weeks or months, increasingly tired, off your food, mildly feverish at times or losing weight, and the back pain has become a painful highlight against this background, you must consult your doctor.

● **Loss of sensation** Widespread numbness and pins and needles in either or both legs may indicate a serious problem, and you must see your doctor. It is possible that a large disc prolapse is damaging the nerves in the spinal canal.

The numbness must be distinguished from the temporary pins and needles caused by sitting or lying awkwardly.

Getting it into perspective
The vast majority of readers should by now have been able to set aside any secret fears, secure in the knowledge that their backache is due to a straightforward mechanical breakdown which will improve with time.

Meanwhile, what should you do? Try to get your problem into perspective. Ask yourself the following questions:
● Is the pain so severe that you need a prescription for strong pain-killers?
● Is it bearable if you find a comfortable position and relax into it?
● After a while in a comfortable position, is it less painful when you move again?
● Are you content to rest and wait for a steady, natural recovery?

There are various useful tips for reducing the pain and improving your ability to move freely, all of which will be discussed later. If, however, your condition does not match up with any of the types of acute episode described in Chapter 4, consult your doctor before attempting to help yourself by trying any of the measures described below.

REST AND RELAXATION

After almost any kind of physical shock to the body, rest is an essential part of first aid. In the first place, it can do no harm when applied for a short time, and secondly it can often do much good. In an acute attack of back pain, lying flat may well be the best course of action for the first few days. It is very important, though, not to rest too long, as this may make recovery slower and could even mean that you never fully recover, as the affected part may stiffen up.

There are a number of advantages in resting the spine by lying down horizontally. You are taking the weight off the joints and discs, which will relieve pain, and may help the damage to heal. When you are sitting or standing, the injured area must still bear its normal load of body weight. Compared with pressure of 100 per cent when the spine is vertical, pressure is only 75 per cent if you lie on your side; when you lie on your back it is reduced to 25 per cent.

In addition, pain often makes muscles seize up in an instinctive protective spasm (if you can't move, you can't be hurt). If the pain is reduced by lying down, the muscles relax, so that pain caused by stiff muscles is relieved.

Rest does not necessarily mean lying down: if the attack is not so painful as to immobilize you, it may be a question of just reducing the level of certain daily activities. Avoid carrying heavy objects, stop doing heavy manual work and try not to drive or to sit at a desk for long periods. All these steps should help to prevent your backache from deteriorating into acute, immobilizing pain.

Relaxation

As you are lying there, you should try to relax as much as you can, both mentally and physically (see page 171 for a simple, practical technique to calm the mind as well as the body). You will not relax physically if you are worrying about the children, finishing the paperwork, or not being a burden to others.

Learn to breathe easily

The key to muscular relaxation is correct breathing. Most of our busy waking life is spent without awareness of how we are breathing. A fixed habit of shallow breathing, tense diaphragm, tight jaw and throat can develop.

When you breathe in, let your mouth stay open in a relaxed way and instead of simply expanding your chest, breathe deeply so that your diaphragm descends and your abdomen rises. If you are relaxed your chest hardly needs to rise at all – it is the diaphragm that should provide the automatic rhythm to breathing. Do not try to breathe in too deeply or too quickly.

Concentrate on exhalation. Let your jaw relax, your mouth fall open and your chest sink when you breathe out.

It often helps to let go with a prolonged and audible sigh.

Imagine the muscles in each part of your body letting go of the tension. Start with the face, then the neck and work downwards. Repeat the process, checking every area.

COMFORTABLE POSITIONS

It is commonly recommended that you should lie flat on your back with a board under the mattress. You need a board only if you have an old bed-base and the springs in your mattress have gone. If you have a good firm base, preferably the floor or wooden slats, and a firm but not too hard mattress, there is no need for a board underneath. The mattress needs to be firm but compressible so that it contours to your shape. A sagging mattress can be bad for your spine.

Keeping your spine horizontal

Lying flat on your back reduces the pressure on your spine to a minimum, but, depending on your injury, it may not be the most comfortable position. The important point is for the spine to be horizontal.

When you are lying on your back, do not use a pillow under your head unless you feel very uncomfortable without one; even then you should use only one pillow, otherwise your spine may flex too much. Special pillows for avoiding neck pain are available (see page 144). If you are lying on your side, put a small pillow between your knees to help keep your spine straight.

Lying on your front, face down, is as good if not better in some situations than lying on your side and is worth a try. However, its effects vary considerably from one person to another. If a disc is protruding towards the back of the spine, this position may be too painful initially. If you have an inflamed or

RESTING YOUR SPINE

Experiment to find the best resting position. There is nothing wrong with lying on your side if this is the most comfortable for you, and, depending on the nature of your disorder, one side may be much more comfortable than the other.

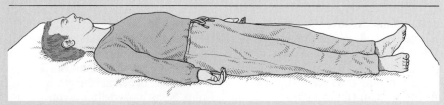

Flat on your back
In this position pressure on the spine is at its minimum, so most back conditions benefit from it, but make sure that your lower back is not arched.

The Fowler position
If you find lying flat on your back uncomfortable, lie with your knees bent at right angles and your legs supported with pillows; this reduces the curve in your lower back.

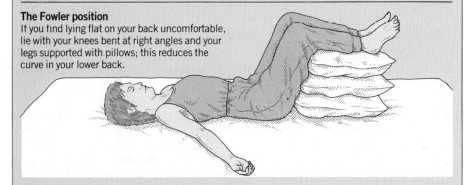

Lying on your side
Place a small pillow between your knees to prevent your hips rotating and twisting your spine.

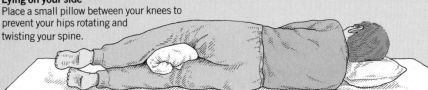

Supporting your neck
Neck pain may be relieved by giving your head extra support at night. Roll up a small towel into a sausage shape, then place it round your neck. This acts as a soft collar and prevents your head lolling to either side.

sprained facet joint, the prone position may also be uncomfortable, and in both disc and facet joint problems the Fowler position, with your legs bent may be the optimum (see page 69). This position gently stretches the lower back, opening the facet joints slightly, and accomodating the protruding disc rather than pinching it, which in turn encourages the protective muscle tension to relax. Over the ensuing days gradually lower your legs by using fewer pillows.

Sitting

Some people find that sitting is the most comfortable position, however the main problem with this is that recovery may be very slow because the pressure on the injured part will then be 150 per cent (see page 139). If you do find it more comfortable to sit up, it is important that you keep your back straight if your pain is caused by a protruding disc. You may be slouching as you sit so that the disc is no longer pressing on a nerve. The weight of your spine will still be pressing down on the disc and preventing it returning to its correct position.

Neck pain

In acute neck pain, you may find that it hurts simply to hold your head up. If so, spend the first day or two lying flat to avoid added stress. When sleeping, tuck a twisted pillow or a rolled and twisted towel round your neck like a thick scarf.

Stay in bed

Once you are committed to a few days' rest, do not compromise by getting up and helping around the house. This will undo all the beneficial effects of rest. Enjoy being looked after if you are fortunate enough to have the help.

To relieve boredom listen to music, read a book, watch television or use the telephone, but do not be tempted into sitting up to play a game or watch television. Stay flat and fix a mirror like a periscope or put the television set high above the bed. Eat your meals lying on your side, or propped up on one elbow.

When you are resting, the only reason you should have for getting up is to go to the toilet and even that is best avoided by the use of a bottle or bed-pan. Most people become constipated if they lie around for more than a few days so to avoid this, eat a high-fibre diet and take laxatives. Do not strain on the toilet.

If walking is too painful, crawl to the bathroom. To stand up, pull yourself up with your arms against some furniture.

PAIN RELIEF

Severe pain causes muscles to go into spasm, which in turn increases your pain (see Chapter 15, Understanding pain). Relief from pain therefore not only makes you more comfortable, it is part of the therapy for back trouble. Try some of the remedies suggested here, but even if your pain is temporarily relieved, do not be tempted to return to your normal activities until your back is completely free of pain and feels strong.

Heat or ice

Both of these are recommended for pain relief. Since heat, in the form of a hot water bottle, is the more comfortable, it is worth trying first. Place the hot water bottle against the most painful part of your back and it will have a soothing effect. Tight muscles may relax just as they do when you sit in a hot bath.

In general, you should avoid baths because, although lying in hot water can relieve the pain, you may be struck with severe pain when you try to get out.

Ice, for example, in the form of a pack of frozen peas wrapped in a thin cloth, or ice cubes crushed in a pack, can be applied over the painful area for 15 minutes every two to three hours, to relieve pain and reduce muscle tension.

Medicines

Try common household pain remedies, such as aspirin, codeine or paracetamol. I tend to favour aspirin, although there is some risk of gastric irritation if it is used for a prolonged period, and you should definitely avoid it if you have had a stomach ulcer. If you take it regularly, (for an adult two tablets every four to six hours for the first four or five days), it will not only relieve your pain but will also reduce any inflammation. This latter effect is most important in those conditions which involve some inflammation, such as facet-joint irritation or swelling around the dural root sleeve. Aspirin may also counter the irritant effect of a protruding disc and can reduce the inflammation caused by local internal bleeding in cases where the muscles, ligaments or joints have been damaged (blood is a tissue irritant when lying outside its normal channels).

In most parts of the world other mild anti-inflammatory agents of proven safety and effectiveness can be bought over the counter in a pharmacy. It is important to realize that these pills are best taken regularly rather than sporadically, since the pain control is much greater when blood levels are maintained.

Massage

This can help to relax muscles as well as to relieve pain, and it is an ideal method to try if you have a willing partner or friend. He or she does not have to be an expert or trained masseur/masseuse to give a soothing but firm massage. He simply needs to have sensitive hands and to be willing and relatively free of tension. This calm and reassuring attitude to touching a friend or partner's body is very comforting. It is important, too, that the person who is being massaged is lying in a comfortable position.

We have both a voluntary and an involuntary response to pain in the spine. A protective muscle action prevents the spinal segments around the source of trouble from moving. This is the involuntary, or reflex, response. The voluntary response involves the individual's reaction to pain and all his fears and anxieties. It produces a more generalized muscular tension. This kind of tension can respond very well to a good massage. For advice on how to give an effective massage, see pages 172 to 173.

Vibrators

There are various electrically powered vibro-massage units which may help.

One kind is a hand-held unit with a smooth rounded cone at one end and a more bulbous surface at the other. The cone-shaped end is used to focus on particular sore nodules in the muscles. The large rounded end is suitable for larger muscle groups. Another type has cushioned, vibrating pads; some models even contain a heating element.

These vibro-massage units are all very easy to use. Place the pad or end on the most painful part of your back and hold it there for a few minutes. Then move on to another area of your back. Most vibrators have a variable frequency control and an intensity or amplitude control, which you can tune to a combination that gives you most relief and comfort. Never place a vibrator directly over a bony area; if a bone is injured in any way, vibrators will not be helpful. Vibrators encourage muscles to relax in much the same way as massage, and stimulate nerve fibres in the skin, thus over-riding the pain messages. They are claimed to improve the condition of the muscles by influencing lymphatic drainage and circulation, but this may be a secondary effect of the pain relief and the relaxation of muscle tension.

Rubs

These include horse liniment, tiger balm, aromatic rubs and modern pharmacological creams. There are two basic types: those with an active pharmacological base, such as aspirin, and those with strongly aromatic or irritant oils.

The former are supposed to work by absorption through the skin into the deeper layers of muscles, but there is little evidence of this, though a small amount may enter the bloodstream.

The counter-irritants, such as "deep heat" or mentholatum, work by creating a burning sensation on the skin, which "distracts" the brain temporarily. You perceive the skin sensation rather than the local muscle or joint pain. (See Chapter 15 for a fuller account of pain perception.) Once the muscle is free of pain, it relaxes of its own accord.

In reality, however, most of the benefit probably comes from the fact that the oils are massaged into the skin. They may give some relief in mild to moderate pain but they are not lasting or effective in swamping more severe pain.

DAY-TO-DAY LIVING

During an acute attack of back pain, your movements will be considerably limited. You will have to adapt yourself to this temporarily restricted lifestyle, and while the pain is severe you should move about as little as possible. When you move, always think before you do anything, to avoid sparking off the pain.

Moving

As soon as you change from a static position, you put your back under fresh stresses and strains. You should start moving as soon as the pain has begun to die down. The tips on the opposite page will help you to change position with the minimum of discomfort.

Clothes

While your back is painful, avoid wearing clothes that are difficult to put on or take off, such as tight jeans. Use slip-on shoes rather than lace-ups if you can. In the box opposite are a few hints to help you dress without hurting your back.

Exercises

After the initial severe pain has subsided (which may vary from 12 to 24 hours to two or three days), it is important to start early mobilizing exercises. These will prevent your back stiffening up, and some are designed specifically to help ease the gel-like nucleus of a disc back towards the centre. Others gently stretch the facet joints and relieve pressure on the spine. They are all described fully in Chapter 14.

Returning to active daily life

Since the majority of people with acute back or neck pain recover spontaneously within one month, the chances are that after a few days you will be feeling like getting up and moving around. It is essential at this stage that you do not jeopardize your progress by ignoring the basic principles of back care (see Chapter 13). The tissues are still in the healing phase and must not be put under excessive strain, even if you feel no pain.

MOVING WITHOUT PAIN

If you sit down carelessly, or bend your back while you are dressing, you will put a lot of unnecessary strain on your lumbar spine. Even getting out of bed could spark off the pain. The advice given below may prevent painful twinges in the joints in your lower back. With practice, these movements will become fluent, and you should continue the habit of moving like this even when your back is not painful.

GETTING OUT OF BED

1 Bring your knees up to about hip level and roll over on to your side.

2 Lower your feet to the floor and use your arms to push yourself up into a sitting position. Reverse this procedure to get back into bed.

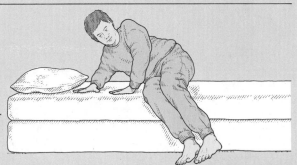

GETTING IN AND OUT OF AN ARMCHAIR

1 Bring your feet as close as you can to the edge of the chair, if possible under the edge. At the same time, bring your buttocks vertically above your feet. Keep your knees at least a shoulder width apart to provide good balance.

2 Keep your spine straight, and place your hands on the arms of the chair.

3 Slowly straighten your legs and push yourself out of the chair with your arms.

4 To sit down in a chair, stand with your back to the chair and your feet a shoulder width apart, close to the edge of the chair. Keep your back straight, and lower yourself slowly. Place your hands on the arms of the chair as soon as you can.

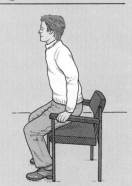

GETTING DRESSED

Whatever the cause of your back pain, these tips will help you to start the day without straining your back. Avoid sitting down and bending over to put your clothes on, as this will strain your back needlessly.

1 Roll your clothes up so that you can put your arms or legs through quickly and easily.

2 Stand on one leg (lean against a wall if necessary) and raise your knee as high as possible to dress your lower half.

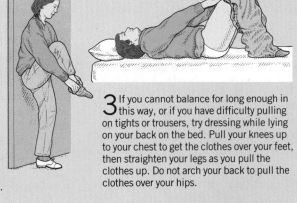

3 If you cannot balance for long enough in this way, or if you have difficulty pulling on tights or trousers, try dressing while lying on your back on the bed. Pull your knees up to your chest to get the clothes over your feet, then straighten your legs as you pull the clothes up. Do not arch your back to pull the clothes over your hips.

6

A professional diagnosis

A proper diagnosis is essential before you can have conventional medical treatment. The person best equipped to start the process is your family doctor: not only does he have access to all the tools of investigation, but he is able to refer you to the appropriate specialist or therapist. In Britain at least, the main drawback about consulting your doctor is that many doctors do not have sufficient time, interest or depth of knowledge about back pain and its causes, and you may not receive as much help as you need.

On the other hand, "alternative" practitioners, such as osteopaths and chiropractors, cannot offer such a variety of investigations. Therefore, if you consult such a practitioner in the first instance, your problem may not be diagnosed properly. You also need to find a practitioner whom you can trust, and whose qualifications are complete. For information on selecting a practitioner, see Useful Addresses, page 187.

Finding a qualified alternative therapist is easier in countries such as the United States, where practitioners such as osteopaths are accepted as part of the general medical system. Ideally, all general practitioners should receive adequate training in the methods of orthopaedic medicine, including examination of joints, diagnosis of disorders in muscles, ligaments, spinal joints and discs, and recognition of conditions best treated by manipulation and massage. It is estimated that as many as a quarter of patients consulting a family doctor would benefit from such treatment.

The pragmatic solution for the time being is that you start with your family doctor – particularly if it is your first attack of back pain – and get the benefit of the doctor's opinion, plus access to further investigations, physiotherapy and medication. If you have been through this stage and it proved unsatisfactory, you are perfectly free to consult any practitioner of your choice, alternative or otherwise, although you may need to approach medical consultants through your doctor, and it is wise to keep your doctor informed.

You should see your family doctor first if you are in severe pain; or if you fall into any of the categories listed on pages 66 to 67. If you wish to consult a practitioner other than your doctor, I would advise the following courses of action, depending on the type and severity of your pain.

● Consult a medical manipulator or an orthopaedic physician, an osteopath, chiropractor, or manipulative physio-therapist if your pain is bearable but is not settling after ten to 14 days, or if you are in a hurry to get better.

● If you are prone to frequent and recur-ring episodes of back or neck pain, go to see a physiotherapist who has received training in Back School methods (see page 91) for prevention of back pain and general care of the back, or consult an orthopaedic physician.

● If you have chronic back pain, go to a specialist in orthopaedics or rheuma-tology, or a Pain Clinic; then if neither can help, consult an orthopaedic physi-cian, an acupuncturist, homeopath or other therapist. (These therapies are discussed in later chapters.)

CONSULTING YOUR DOCTOR

When you go to your doctor, he will probably want you to answer the follow-ing questions. Try to answer them as fully and clearly as possible, to help him make an accurate diagnosis.

● What were you doing when the pain first started?

● Did the pain come on suddenly or did it build up gradually?

● Where do you feel the pain, and where does it radiate to?

● What is the pain like – sharp, dull, heavy, burning?

● Is it constant?

● What positions or movements relieve it, and which aggravate it?

● Do you feel any patches of numbness or pins and needles?

● Have you had similar attacks before?

● What kind of job do you do?

● What daily actions involve your back?

Describing your pain

It is important to describe the type of pain you are experiencing, as well as its intensity, since this will help the doctor to make an accurate diagnosis. There are a large number of adjectives that can express the quality and severity of pain. Some of these describe the physical sensation, for example, pulsating, shoot-ing, stabbing, sharp. Perhaps your pain is gnawing, pulling, burning, searing or stinging. You may find that words reflecting the emotional feeling associ-ated with the pain are more descriptive, such as tiring, wretched, sickening, miserable, frightful. Other words evalu-ate the overall intensity of the pain, for example dreadful, vicious, unbearable, terrible or torturing.

Different types of pain have different causes. A general, dull ache is often caused by tense muscles or irritation deep within the spinal joints, while a sharp, shooting pain may be caused by a pinched nerve and – as with sciatica and brachialgia – it may not be felt at the site of injury. A sharp but clearly defined pain which does not spread to any other sites comes from pinched tissues such as the skin or the lining on a bone. A dif-fused, burning sensation is often caused by a disturbance of the sympathetic nerves, which control involuntary, sub-conscious functions such as circulation and sweating. These nerves do not control any voluntary actions, so you would not notice any weakness accom-panying the pain.

Preliminary treatment

The doctor will give you a thorough physical examination, and he should be able to make at least a preliminary diagnosis. He will almost certainly re-commend rest in bed, probably with a board under the mattress, though if

PHYSICAL EXAMINATION

When you have answered all the doctor's questions she will give you a physical examination. She will probably ask you to undress to your underwear, so that she can observe your back as you move and bend, and feel your spine for tender areas.

The doctor will look at your posture as you stand up, and will ask you to bend forwards, backwards and to each side, telling her as you do so exactly at which point the pain is made worse.

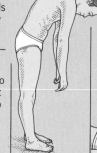

You will be asked to lie down on your back, and the doctor will raise each leg up straight until you feel pain.

She will test your knee and ankle reflexes and your foot responses, and perhaps will use a pin to detect any numbness of the skin. She might test the strength of your leg muscles by asking you to pull your foot up while she holds it down.

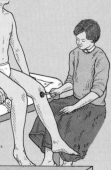

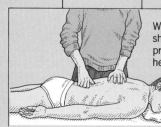

While you lie on your front, she will feel for tenderness by pressing on your spine with her hands.

your bed is firm you may not need a board (see page 68). He may prescribe some pain-killers, anti-inflammatory drugs and muscle relaxants or a combination of these. He may also give you a sheet of "do's and don'ts" for backache.

Muscle relaxants and some pain-killers may affect your level of alertness. Do not be alarmed if you feel drowsy while taking them, but if you do, avoid driving and any other activities requiring high levels of concentration. In general you will probably sleep quite well, but do not mix your medication with alcohol. Your doctor may also prescribe a stool-softener since some of the strong pain-killers, particularly the narcotic drugs, might cause constipation.

If you are in severe pain, you will probably need a strong analgesic to take regularly. Unfortunately, a practitioner who has not suffered from a bad back or acute sciatica may not appreciate the level of pain you are experiencing, and may not give adequate pain relief. Do not be afraid to ask for stronger pain-killers: in general, there is no need to fear that you may become addicted to the pain-killer, even if it is an opiate derivative. If you have any worries about addiction, you should discuss them with your doctor.

If you experience recurrent episodes of back pain, and your job entails lifting or carrying heavy objects, your doctor will advise you to take time off work until you have fully recovered. Alternatively, if the attacks are becoming more severe and prolonged, he may discuss the possibility of returning to lighter duties or even changing jobs.

FURTHER INVESTIGATIONS

Your doctor may be more concerned to investigate if the pain is very severe or prolonged, or if it is recurring very frequently. The first and most likely set of investigations will be:

● Full blood count
● Erythrocyte (red blood cell) sedimentation rate, ESR
● X-ray.

Blood tests

From a single blood sample taken in the surgery, the doctor can take a blood count and test the ESR. The full blood count, which discloses the numbers of the various types of blood cell, may reveal infection or anaemia, indicating that there may be an underlying disease.

The ESR is a general indicator of chronic inflammation, infection, or a tumour. In inflammatory diseases of the spine, the rate at which the red blood cells settle is usually raised. Examples of such diseases include ankylosing spondylitis, rheumatoid arthritis, which should be obvious from the other joints involved, and inflammation of the sacroiliac joint, which is associated in most cases with inflammation of the bowel and other systemic disorders.

X-rays

The standard set of X-rays for the neck and lower spine involves three separate views taken with you lying down. The X-rays may reveal specific causes for the pain, such as a fracture, spondylolisthesis/spondylolysis (see page 54), a tumour or infection or advanced ankylosing spondylitis (see page 63). They may show degenerative changes, including disc narrowing, osteophyte formation (see page 59) or narrowing of the foramina (the gaps between the vertebrae), which may not be connected with your pain.

The soft tissues, which include muscle, ligament, cartilage, and disc, do not show up on X-rays, and since these structures are usually causing the pain, X-rays often provide only negative information. In 95 per cent of patients, X-rays exclude the possibility of bone damage or serious bone disease, but do not show the real cause of the trouble.

In people over 30 years old degenerative joint disease may show up, but this may not be significant to the cause of pain. If there are relevant degenerative changes showing on the X-ray, your doctor will probably interpret these to you as "wear and tear" on the spine.

CONSULTING A SPECIALIST

If your attack is not settling after four to six weeks of conventional treatment and X-rays show either no bony cause or just simple degenerative changes, your doctor may refer you to a specialist – usually an orthopaedic or rheumatology specialist. Alternatively, he might send you to a physiotherapy department for treatment. In some regions of the United Kingdom there are orthopaedic physicians who deal with such problems.

Your family doctor will send a letter to the specialist stating your medical history, the nature of your complaint, any drugs he has prescribed, and your progress. He will also include the results of any blood tests or X-rays that you have already had.

Most specialists want to see how your spine looks on X-ray. Some will want to take views of your spine bent fully backwards, forwards and sideways, to determine whether one of your vertebrae is shifting slightly. If there is an unusual shadow in or near the bone, they will want closer and more focused views of that particular section: these are called tomograms or CT scans (see page 81).

Depending on the results of your X-rays, the specialist may then order a variety of traditional treatments, including physiotherapy, traction, a spinal support, a plaster jacket or further rest in bed. If, however, you have been in severe pain for many weeks, have lost much time off work, and show clear signs of nerve damage to one or more of the sciatic nerves, the specialist may be inclined to take more urgent action.

SPECIALIST INVESTIGATIONS

If you have been suffering from chronic back pain and the specialist suggests that you have any of the following investigations, do not be put off by the fact that some of them entail injections. Even if there is a certain amount of pain or discomfort involved in the investigation, this may be offset by a local anaesthetic. In the long run, anything that will help you to find out what is really wrong and indicate how your problem can be solved has to be well worth trying. For most of these tests, you will have to attend the out-patient's department of a hospital, but for a myelogram (see opposite) you will need to stay in hospital for a day or so.

Blood tests

In addition to the full blood count and the ESR, the specialist may also want to check your blood levels of calcium, phosphate, alkaline phosphatase enzyme and vitamin D: if these are abnormal, you may have a bone disease.

If the specialist suspects inflammation, such as ankylosing spondylitis, he may arrange for you to have another blood test, known as HLA-B27, which tests for a tissue marker found in 93 per cent of sufferers from ankylosing spondylitis.

Specialized X-rays

If the first batch of X-rays did not show anything useful, further more specialized X-rays may be considered. These will include dynamic studies, which are X-ray stills taken to show you bending forwards, backwards and sideways as far as you can manage, with the aim of showing whether any segments of the spine are not moving enough or are unstable and consequently too mobile.

The specialist may also want to see inclined plane views, for which you must lie on a tilting table. This type of X-ray is useful for delineating individual vertebra and disc spaces and for post-operative assessment.

If you have some spinal deformity and low back or leg pain, an X-ray may be taken of your whole spine rather than just the visibly deformed section, since an obvious deformity can rise to compensate for a hidden deformity somewhere else and this will show up on an X-ray of the full length of the spine. For example, a hunched upper back may develop to compensate for a less obvious curve in the lower back.

Standing X-rays, rather than X-rays taken when you are lying down, may show that a vertebra has slipped out of line, forwards or backwards (see spondylolisthesis, page 54).

Myelogram

This is a type of X-ray in which a dye is injected into the spinal canal. It is sometimes called radiculography, and is generally carried out only if a specialist is considering surgery. Myelography, and

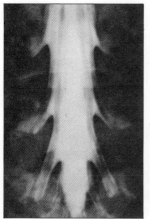
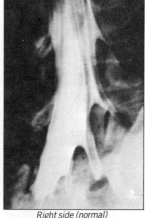
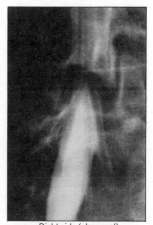

Back (normal)   *Right side (normal)*   *Right side (abnormal)*

Myelogram Myelograms of a normal spine (above left and centre) show the spinal cord and the nerve root sleeves filled with dye, which appears white.

In the myelogram on the right, a prolapsed disc blocks the dye, and shows up as a dark indentation on the spinal canal.

electromyography (see right), are both particularly useful in determining accurately the exact level of disc disease.

For a myelogram you will be admitted to hospital for 24 hours or for as long as may be needed for the side-effects, which can include headache, nausea and vomiting in some 10 to 12 per cent of people, to settle down.

Under a local anaesthetic, dye is injected into the spinal canal via a direct lumbar puncture through the protective dural sheath which lines the inside of the canal. This is done while you lie on a table that tilts so that you can be tilted down, causing the dye to run into the dural sleeves around the nerves in the lower back, or upwards for the upper back. During this procedure, X-rays are taken from the front and both sides to detect "filling defects", where the disc or some other obstruction is encroaching on the dural sheath. It is an uncomfortable procedure lasting about 20 to 30 minutes, but the local anaesthetic prevents it becoming too painful.

In Great Britain and the United States iodized oil was once used, but this has now been superseded by water-soluble contrast dye. This is because the oil-based views were found to be less accurate in some cases, and also because the oil sometimes caused painful arachnoiditis (see page 64).

Electromyography

This technique is used as a diagnostic tool to measure the activity of various muscle groups when your spine is at rest or moving. It identifies which nerve root has been damaged, by revealing a deterioration in the activity of the muscles linked to that root. This gives further clues on the location of a protruding disc. Electromyography entails inserting find gauge needles into a muscle in the leg, foot or calf and detecting the electrical impulses coming from it. The procedure takes about 30 minutes. There are no side-effects and the only pain is a slight pricking, rather like a vaccination.

Epidural venography

A recent development, this may prove to be a useful adjunct to myelography. It is a time-consuming procedure, though you can have it done as a day-patient. It is not comfortable, but not especially painful either. A dye is injected through the femoral vein in the groin into a vein going up the lower back. On X-ray, this shows up the epidural vertebral veins, which form a regular lozenge-shaped pattern applied to the backs of the vertebrae and discs. If this pattern is distorted, you may be suffering from a disc prolapse.

Epidurography

This is another form of X-ray, in which a dye is injected into the epidural space – the area between the bony walls of the spinal canal and the dural sheath – with the aim of showing up any protrusion of a disc. It is not painful, and takes about 30 minutes. The disadvantage of this method is that after surgery or recurrent disc prolapses, the epidural space may be obliterated by scar tissue and will therefore not show up clearly.

Discography

This test may be suggested if you do not have typical patterns of pain. The procedure can take quite a long time. You will be given a local anaesthetic, then a small amount of dye is injected via a long needle inserted into the centre of the disc that is suspected of causing your symptoms. It can be painful, and you will be asked to report any symptoms provoked by this procedure. The investigator compares the provoked symptoms to the usual symptoms. Discography can identify a suspected disc prolapse if a myelogram has not shown anything. It identifies disc degeneration, and is useful when back or leg pain recurs after surgery for disc prolapse.

Facet arthrography

This determines whether pain in the back, hip, groin or leg is caused by inflammation or osteoarthritis of the facet joints. The test takes about 30 minutes, and may be slightly painful. Under local anaesthetic a small amount of dye is injected into the joint to verify that the joint is fitting together properly as it should. If the local anaesthetic then relieves the symptoms and signs, which may include pain in the back or leg, limited straight leg raising and sluggish tendon reflexes, a therapeutic injection can be given (see page 108).

Bone scan

A solution containing a minute quantity of radioactive material in injected into a vein and is taken up by bone so that hyperactive areas (areas which are renewing themselves too quickly) can be identified within a few hours. Increased bone turnover can occur due to a variety

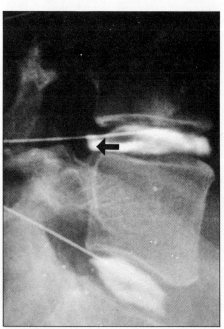

Discography
The middle disc is ruptured, allowing the dye to run from the nucleus of the disc through the outer layers into the spinal canal.

of causes, such as a healing fracture, infection and tumour. The pictures obtained reveal "hot spots" up to three months before they would be detected by routine X-rays. This procedure is painless and free of side-effects, but takes several hours, since you have to wait for two or three hours between the injection and the scan.

CT scan

Also known as the 'Cat scan' or computed tomography, this has come into operation over the last ten years and represents a tremendous advance in the investigation of spinal disorders. At the moment, it is available in only a few major hospitals. It is entirely painless and takes 20 to 30 minutes. It is basically a sophisticated X-raying technique that can take "slices" or sectional views throughout the length and breadth of the spine and provide three-dimensional information. It will show not just the bony tissue but also soft tissues such as muscles and adjacent visceral organs such as the stomach, gall-bladder and liver. It can also identify the position of the bones and the facet joints and their relationship to the spinal canal and the gaps in the vertebrae more accurately than a conventional X-ray. Combining this with myelography allows a closer study of the nerve tissue and the processes affecting it.

Ultrasound scan

This technique involves the reflection of ultrasound echoes. The more dense the structure, such as bone, the greater the echoes. It is a risk-free and painless investigation lasting only 15 minutes. A metal scanning head is applied to the back, and a gel may be spread on the skin to help transmission of the ultrasound waves. In the spine it is used to measure the width of the spinal canal, and so can detect those people with narrow canals who are at greater risk of developing back pain or sciatica. It may also help orthopaedic surgeons who are planning particular kinds of operations, such as spinal fusion (see page 114), to prevent certain complications.

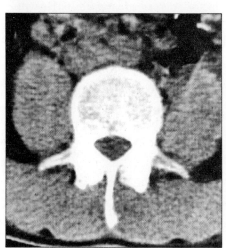 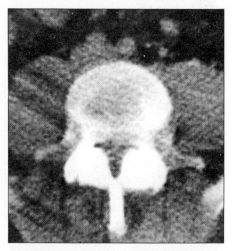

CT scan (Computed tomography)
A cross-section of the vertebra shows up on the CT scans, with the spinal canal and the processes all clearly visible. Damage to muscles, discs and ligaments, as well as to bones, will show up. The spine on the right has an abnormally narrow canal.

7
Physiotherapy

With its combined approach of exercise, massage and manipulation (the manual adjustment of joints), physiotherapy can be one of the most effective forms of treatment for back pain. It is generally preferable to surgery, and in many cases more beneficial than taking drugs.

Your first appointment will probably be arranged through your doctor after he has made a diagnosis, since a physiotherapist cannot order X-rays or certain other investigations. Although all qualified physiotherapists have about three to four years of hospital training, their techniques vary widely according to where they have trained. Your doctor will refer you to the most suitable department in your local hospital or to an individual therapist. If you have already received treatment from a physiotherapist and the problem recurs, there is no harm in consulting the physiotherapist directly.

CONSULTING A PHYSIOTHERAPIST

The physiotherapist will make a thorough assessment of the spine and its related functions before starting treatment. Many are unwilling to accept a patient with a spinal problem without an X-ray, but the importance of X-rays as a screening procedure for low back pain is declining as assessment through physical examination improves, so a physiotherapist who does not request an X-ray may simply be more confident.

Diagnosis
As with all medical consultations, diagnosis starts from the moment you walk in the room. The physiotherapist will take a full history of your symptoms and will then examine you. He will observe the way you walk, stand and sit, and will ask you to bend forwards, backwards and sideways. His preliminary examination will be very similar to the doctor's described on page 76. He will also feel your whole back, testing the movement of individual segments, and feeling for any tender or tense spots in the muscles.

PRELIMINARY TREATMENT
A physiotherapist's tools are his hands: he may be able to treat the problem in your spine using simply massage and manipulation. All physiotherapists are trained in some methods of manipulation and massage, although techniques may differ between individual therapists. The Maitlands method (see opposite) is one of the most common. There is also an increasing amount of electronic equipment available to therapists, for both treatment and diagnosis, and this is described in the next section.

Massage

This is more than just a pleasurable, relaxing ancillary treatment. It can be therapeutic when applied to taut muscles and, since it relaxes you, it is an important preliminary to manipulation.

Massage given by a physiotherapist is likely to include deep transverse friction massage, in which he massages with his fingers across the fibres of ligaments and muscles to break up scar tissue, improve blood supply and increase mobility. He may also use connective tissue massage, a technique only recently developed. It involves stretching the skin by drawing the finger tip over certain pathways to stimulate blood flow and encourage the muscles to relax. This method makes use of the many interconnections between the nerves supplying the skin and those supplying the muscles in the same region. It may work through various reflex pathways in the spinal cord.

Other methods of massage include stroking, kneading, vibratory movements and petrissage (pinching and stretching adjacent muscle areas), all of which help to reduce fluid in the muscle tissue. A good physiotherapist will have developed his own techniques.

Mobilization

All physiotherapists in Britain now learn and use the Maitlands method to mobilize spinal and other joints. The method entails gentle rhythmic movements of a spinal joint near the limit of its normal range of movement in order to stretch the ligaments. No thrust is made beyond the normal "joint range" This means that if it feels painful, you can resist at any time simply by tightening your muscles, so one of the advantages of this method is that you still feel in control of what is being done to you. It is also gentler than some techniques and there is less mystique and therefore less prejudice amongst orthodox circles. However, it is probably slower and less effective than manipulation.

Heat and ice

Almost any back pain may temporarily benefit from heat and exercises, and

---

MAITLANDS MOBILIZATION

This method of mobilization is commonly used by physiotherapists to flex joints and increase their range of movement. The techniques are graded from one to five, to describe how much force is used: the higher the number, the greater the force.

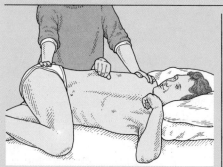

Rotational mobilization
This rotates the spine to the right, putting grade 4 rotational force on the third lumbar vertebra.

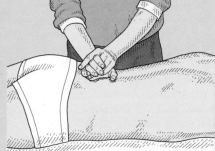

Central mobilization
By pressing down on the spine, the therapist mobilizes the fifth lumbar vertebra with grade 4 force.

on some occasions physiotherapists use ice. I have already discussed the use of these as a self-help measure (see page 70) and there seems very little point in a specialist applying further heat therapy in whatever form – whether he uses infra-red, peat-packs, wax-baths, hot pads or a hot water bottle. All forms will have a temporarily soothing effect, helping to relax tense muscles and encouraging local blood flow. They may decrease joint stiffness.

ELECTRONIC EQUIPMENT

Unfortunately, a number of medically trained people believe that massage and manipulation are unscientific. Their opinions have encouraged some physiotherapists to neglect these techniques in favour of using electronic equipment, in order to win the approval of the more conventional scientists. However, I strongly believe that massage and manipulation can be very beneficial, and that modern electronic devices often give only temporary relief.

Ultrasound

One of the most popular therapeutic tools of the physiotherapist, ultrasound is used to treat soft tissue injuries, such as damage to a muscle, ligament, tendon or joint capsule. It can also be used to treat trigger point phenomena (see page 49) by encouraging the localized contractions of the muscles to relax. It is used to treat injured muscles, but these are not the main cause of backache.

This treatment is very popular in sports injuries units and can be used to drive a solution of anti-inflammatory cream or cortisone through the skin to settle inflammation in the facet joints.

Ultrasound consists of high frequency soundwaves created by passing an electric current through a crystal. These are then focused directly on to the painful tissue through a round metal "head" by the physiotherapist. A gel is spread on your skin to help the transmission of the waves through the skin.

The intensity and penetration of the ultrasonic beam can be controlled by the physiotherapist by altering the frequency of the wave. The treatment is normally entirely painless without any sensation whatsoever. The physiotherapist can select either a continuous or a pulse transmission. The latter is used more often because it generates less heat. The only risk from ultrasound arises if a continuous beam is focused on a fresh muscle injury which is still bleeding. In this case further bleeding may be encouraged. If the ultrasound waves are applied directly over a bony surface and held there for any length of time, it may cause intense pain, due to reflection off the surface of the bone, but the risk of this is minimal with a skilled user.

You will be given ultrasound treatment on the physiotherapist's couch with the relevant part of your back exposed. Relief from pain will not be immediate, but it is normal to give a course of two or three sessions a week over a few weeks.

Although ultrasound has been used for many years, research into its effectiveness has often produced rather inconclusive results because it is hard to be sure of an accurate diagnosis in back problems and the healing process is equally hard to quantify. Recent studies, however, suggest that it promotes healing by speeding up the different phases of the inflammatory and repair processes in the affected body cells.

Short wave diathermy

This is an electromagnetic wave of high frequency that can promote a healing action on the tissues. It will reduce swelling, stabilize cell membranes and stimulate blood flow. The combination of these factors results in muscle relaxation, decreased joint stiffness and a reduction of pain. To prevent the tissues overheating, the short wave can also be given in a pulsed dosage, which allows the tissues to cool down between pulses. This treatment has been used to heal non-united fractures, suggesting that its effects are more far-reaching than those of straightforward heat treatment.

A painless process, diathermy is given as you lie on the therapist's couch with the relevant part of your back exposed. You will feel better immediately, but this improvement may not last, so you will probably need two or three treatments a week for several weeks. There are no side-effects, particularly since the newest machines automatically give out a pulsed wave which has no deep heating effect. This allows treatment to be given soon after the injury, even if there is still some local bleeding.

Interferential therapy

This is another form of electrotherapy in which a low frequency "interference" wave is produced where two medium-frequency alternating currents coincide.

The physiotherapist can vary the frequency of the interference wave very accurately anywhere between one and 150 cycles a second according to whether he wants to influence the activity of the nerves, muscles, or blood vessels. This therapy helps to reduce inflammation in joints or muscles and has a good, but temporary, pain-relieving action. It can also help non-united fractures to heal.

Interferential therapy is sometimes applied through damp sponges covering electrodes, but it may also be given using suction caps. You will experience a "fizzy" sensation from the electric current and your muscles may twitch involuntarily during treatment if the lower frequency ranges are used. The pain relief may be immediate but unfortunately often lasts only a short while; the treatment has to be given over a course of two or three sessions a week for a few weeks. There are no known side-effects. Interferential therapy is very much in vogue in all physiotherapy departments, although there is little evidence as to its long-term value.

Transcutaneous nerve stimulation

This treatment, TNS, is used to help people in severe pain. An electrical current is passed between two surface electrodes attached to the skin at the points of maximum pain. The stream of impulses blocks the transmission of pain up your spine and therefore inhibits perception in the brain. TNS is used in pain clinics throughout the world and is discussed on page 183.

TRACTION

This method of treatment has been used for many centuries. There are diagrams and descriptions of traction apparatus dating from the time of Hippocrates, and even earlier in the Far East. Over the last 50 years or so, traction has been used to pull the spinal joints apart very gently. This enables the muscles in the back to relax fully, and reduces pressure within the disc, allowing disc bulges to recede. Stretching the spine in this way is also beneficial if your facet joints have been irritated through the spine being compressed by the weight of your body when you stand up. All this can relieve pain and even accelerate recovery.

Despite the strong association between the physical effects of traction and common causes of back pain, studies have not produced any dramatic findings so far, although traction to the cervical spine for neck pain has been shown to be valuable and is commonly used in physiotherapy departments.

If traction is applied properly, using chest and pelvic harnesses on a lumbar traction table, the only discomfort you may experience will be due to the tightness of the harnesses. However, if you have been in traction for 20 minutes or so, you might feel painful twinges as it is being released. If you experence pain as traction is being put on and increased, tell the therapist to stop at once. This may indicate that the protrusion is being pushed harder against the nerve root, particularly if the pain is worse in your leg, and traction is therefore an unsuitable form of treatment for you.

Traction is best given daily if possible so that its cumulative effects can then accelerate recovery. You may feel immediate pain relief once you are put on traction, and although the pain might return partially or even completely, it will be reduced by subsequent treatments. Alternatively, it may be a week before you begin to feel any benefits . from the treatment. If your condition is not improving after two weeks, it is unlikely that you can expect relief from this therapy.

Inversion therapy

There are new variations on the theme of traction: inversion therapy looks the most natural and promising. Various machines now on the market enable you to treat yourself at home or even at work

simply by strapping your ankles to a tilt-frame and swinging backwards – upside down. Inversion therapy is useful in a similar range of back conditions to those treated by horizontal traction.

Once you have become accustomed to the blood rushing to your head, inversion traction feels very comfortable. Unlike horizontal traction, there are no tight chest or pelvic harnesses restricting your breathing or circulation. You can operate the machine yourself simply by moving your arms and you can use it as often as you like, when you like, in your own home.

Muscles relax quite quickly in the fully inverted position, and the length of the spine measurably increases after only a few minutes. Some of this lengthening effect is gained from reabsorption of fluid into the centre of the disc, which

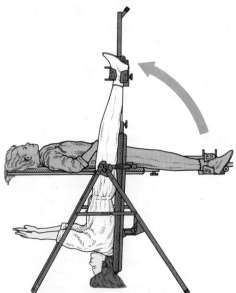

Inversion traction
To use this equipment, you strap your ankles to the tilting frame and lean back. When you bring your arms above your head, you swing backwards until you are upside down. To swing yourself upright again, simply put your hands down at your sides.

nourishes the disc cartilage. Used over a long period, this may delay the degenerative process that occurs due to "drying out", though so far there is no firm evidence to prove this theory. The remaining effect is probably due to improved posture. Inversion therapy may also aid drainage of the veins in the spinal canal, reducing congestion and speeding up the healing process.

In Britain relatively few hospital departments use this form of traction but quite a few private practitioners and physiotherapists have the equipment. In the United States it is more widely available as a form of treatment. If your doctor or physiotherapist decides that it would be suitable for you, he will supervise the first one or two sessions and, provided there is no complication, you may well be able to take the apparatus home and use it at your convenience.

Since back pain is characteristically a recurring problem and the disc degenerates with age, there is a case for recommending the use of a portable inversion traction machine on a regular basis – say, ten to 15 minutes a day – at home.

Although the treatment is completely safe provided you do not suffer from raised blood pressure, a history of strokes or glaucoma (raised pressure in the eyeball), I would not advise anyone to invest in this equipment before consulting their doctor or physiotherapist.

Continuous traction in bed

This is given to people with severe disc protrusions and sciatica rather than for other less painful causes of acute back pain. It involves a stay in hospital and is usually arranged by a specialist, but a physiotherapist is involved in setting up the treatment. The head of the bed is tilted downwards and a weight hung on the end of a rope over a pulley at the foot. Since this provides very little real force on your lower back, most realists admit that it is no more than an effective way of enforcing bedrest. Resting the spine for 24 hours a day may relieve the pain, but it is uncomfortable. You are not allowed to get up to eat or even to fulfil daily bodily functions. You may have difficulty in passing urine normally, and constipation is common – often a combined result of the pain and immobility. It will be treated with muscle relaxants and stool-softeners.

If there is no improvement after two weeks, it is unlikely that any can be expected and you may need to have a myelogram (see page 78) with a view to surgery (see Chapter 10).

Neck Traction

As with bed traction, a physiotherapist will set the traction up. If you have severe pain in your arm caused by a disc in your neck pressing on a nerve, you may feel some relief with neck traction. You will normally be treated in bed, propped up slightly, with a halter – usually made of leather or canvas with woollen padding for comfort – round your neck. The halter is attached via a rope pulley to a weight hanging behind the head end of the bed. You may also be given neck traction sitting up, as a day patient.

Your pain might be so severe that the doctor prescribes very strong painkillers (morphine derivatives) combined with strong sedation. Fortunately, this very severe pain lasts only for a few weeks at the most, unless it has been caused by violent injury to the upper arm resulting in the nerve root being torn off the spinal cord.

Autotraction

Developed in Sweden, this method allows you to be in greater control and to adjust the angle of horizontal traction in

AUTOTRACTION

By holding on to the frame at the top of the couch and pushing the frame at your feet away from you, you can maintain the ideal degree of traction for your spine. The head and foot of the couch can slope up and down, and the therapist will arrange the angle of the two sections to achieve localized traction at the damaged segment.

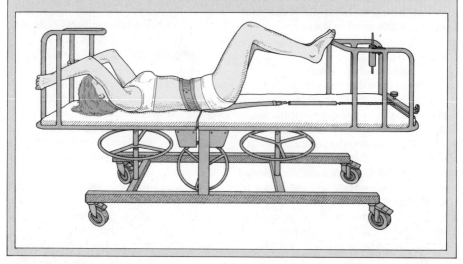

three planes. It is used in the treatment of lower back pain and sciatica caused by disc prolapse.

You will lie on a special couch which has a movable frame at the foot. This frame can slide up and down the length of the couch, so you can push it down with your feet as you lie on the couch. A harness round your hips is attached to the frame by a strap, thus when you push the frame away from you, you put your spine under traction. In this way you can choose the degree of traction yourself. It is always closely supervised by a physiotherapist or practitioner.

Autotraction is reported to give good results and may save a few people from surgery. As in the case of inversion therapy, the inventors of this treatment claim that it may delay disc degeneration.

COLLARS AND CORSETS

A painful back or neck may need some extra support, so a physiotherapist might give you a collar or a corset to wear temporarily. These can relieve acute pain and speed up your recovery, though doctors disagree over how beneficial they are. A corset reduces pressure on your spine by supporting your abdomen, and although it is supposed to restrict movement, some research suggests that your lower spine bends even more if you wear a corset which comes high up your back. A collar helps to support your head and therefore reduces pressure on your neck.

As well as giving your back or neck some support, a collar or corset can also keep it warm, stimulate the nerve ends in the skin which are very sensitive to pressure (an effect similar to massage), remind you to be careful how you move or bend, and help your muscles to relax. You may not like the idea of a collar or corset if it is offered, but it may well provide short-term relief and help to prevent a relapse.

Cervical collars

Collars are frequently used to relieve acutely painful neck conditions. Soft collars are usually made of foam fastened with Velcro, while hard collars are made from a stiffer synthetic material.

Whether your painful neck has developed suddenly on waking one morning or is the result of a whiplash injury (see page 48), a supportive collar will often relieve the pain by restricting your neck movements and helping to support your head. This is only a temporary measure to allow inflammation or bruising around the spinal joints to settle down; you may not need to wear the collar all the time, and you probably won't have to wear it for more than a fortnight.

If you are over the age of about 55, and suffer from chronic neck pain due to severe degenerative changes, it may be suggested that you wear a hard collar during the day permanently, but there are very few people who need such drastic measures.

The vertebral artery, which travels up the neck through a bony canal created by the vertebrae on either side, may be narrowed or compressed in certain positions when you turn your head or stretch your neck. This brings on sudden giddiness and occasionally even blackouts when you look up, turn round, or work with your arms held up, for example, when hanging up washing, or painting a ceiling. This is called the vertebro-basilar syndrome and is partly an effect of the furring and hardening of the arteries which tend to occur with age. If you have this generalized disease of the circulation, combined with narrowing of the vertebral canal in the neck, you may need to control the symptoms by wearing a hard collar all the time to restrict neck movements.

COLLARS AND CORSETS

Most corsets and collars these days are made of a combination of canvas and elastic, foam or neoprene, depending on the amount of flexibility they are intended to provide. There are various kinds of corset — short, long, light and flexible, heavy and ribbed, with or without thoracic bands, lateral uprights and sacral extensions — and a range of sizes to use "off the peg". A more rigid corset can be made specially for you.

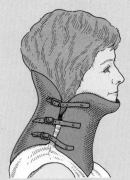

Cervical collar (left)
This stiff collar supports the head, taking weight off the neck, and prevents neck movement.

Spinal corset (right)
The corset covers the buttocks and extends up over the lower ribs. It is important that a corset fits exactly, in order to support the spine while allowing you to sit comfortably. If you need one for long-term use it can be tailored exactly to your shape.

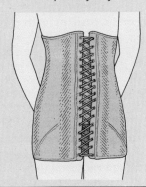

BRACES AND CASTS FOR SCOLIOSIS

Non-surgical treatment of scoliosis depends on the amount of curvature. If the curve is very slight, causing no discomfort and minimal deformity, then it may not be necessary to treat the condition. Traction and bending exercises (see pages 85 and 159) improve flexibility and posture, though they do not prevent the development of the curve. They are helpful in mild scoliosis as well as in slightly more severe cases needing braces. Exercises are also recommended to increase flexibility before surgery.

Braces are commonly used to treat more pronounced curves. They are prescribed and fitted by orthopaedic surgeons rather than physiotherapists. They are normally worn for 23 hours a day and removed only for bathing or any prescribed exercises. Once you stop growing or the curve has improved, they can be worn for reduced periods of time.

Babies with scoliosis may be put into plastercast braces with pressure pads inside and a window cut in the concave side to allow the ribs to grow normally.

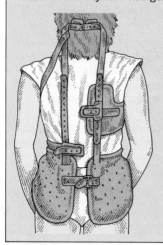

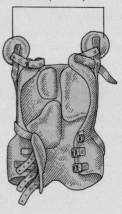

Shoulder pressure pads

Milwaukee brace (left)
This is shown fitted to a patient whose lumbar spine curves to the left, while her thoracic spine curves to the right. The pad over her right shoulder blade is counteracted by the sling under her left arm, to correct the curve of the thoracic spine. The pad over the left side of her waist should straighten her lumbar spine.

Low profile brace (right)
This brace has pads on the inside, positioned to correct the curve of the spine. Supports for the shoulders can be attached if the spine is also rotated.

Corsets

Spinal corsets are used to help treat a wide variety of different back problems. Physiotherapists tend to recommend wearing a corset only as a short-term measure, perhaps for a few weeks after recovering from an acute episode of back pain to enable you to go back to work without risking an early relapse. Very few people are in favour of any long-term use because your spinal joints may become stiff.

OTHER TREATMENTS

The physiotherapist will probably give you advice on posture and the lifting and handling techniques outlined on page 145. He may recommend a course on back care (see Back Schools, opposite) and teach you some of the therapeutic exercises given in Chapter 14.

Some types of back pain are eased by performing gentle stretching and bending exercises in warm water.

Hydrotherapy
Traditionally, rich people sought relief from their aches and pains in health

spas with warm water springs or special minerals. The common ingredient of these treatments is the weightless effect of floating in water; what goes into the water, whether it is salt, mud or sulphur, is probably of minor importance.

Most large hospital physiotherapy departments have a pool for supervised treatment, as do well-supplied private clinics. This is a beneficial treatment for many forms of muscle and joint injury. You can do exercises to strengthen and stretch muscles, while the water supports you and reduces pressure on your joints. Flexibility and mobility can be achieved without risk of exceeding the "normal" range of movement, because the resistance offered by the water restricts your actions. Swimming, too, can have a definite therapeutic effect so long as you do not arch your back while doing the breast stroke in an attempt to keep your head above water.

The Back School approach

This was first developed in Sweden about 15 years ago and is now used in varying forms in Britain, Europe, the United States and Australia. It is not appropriate if you have acute back pain because its purpose is to help those with a long-term back problem. Every Back School differs but the main ingredients of treatment are:

● Postural advice – in standing, sitting and lying
● Specific muscle strengthening exercises for the muscles of the abdomen, back and legs
● Hydrotherapy
● Education– the mechanics of the spine, its anatomy and its physiology; lifting and handling techniques; ergonomics (choosing tools, equipment, furniture and the shape, size and weight of loads to minimize strain on the spine)
● Confidence building.

The main advantages of attending a Back School are that it offers a comprehensive back care programme which includes a thorough clinical examination; a functional assessment to see how you manage everyday tasks; appropriate therapeutic treatment; group classes. This programme is combined with follow-up treatment and support from a team of experts, which may include orthopaedic specialists, psychologists, and specialists in vocational treatment.

A study of its effectiveness has shown that symptoms tend to clear up sooner after Back School treatment. Less time is lost from work by those who attend a Back School, and due to the emphasis on improving general fitness, many participants increase the amount of exercise that they take after going through a Back School.

A growing number of physiotherapy departments now offer something along these lines, although unfortunately trimmed and cut down. In some cases this may amount to no more than an exercise class for back patients, though this can hardly be called a Back School when it omits important factors such as a thorough clinical assessment of each individual's condition.

For long-term results, there is no doubt that improving your posture and learning proper lifting and handling techniques, coupled with adaptation of your working environment, are paramount. Unfortunately, most businesses and factories are still unaware of the importance of work conditions in preventing backache and other disorders.

Neck Schools would probably be just as beneficial and some have now opened in Sweden. The approach is similar to that of the Back School, with its emphasis on helping people with chronic complaints to learn how to live with their problem.

8
Manipulation

More and more doctors are now offering manipulation as a viable alternative to conventional treatment for back pain, and an increasing number of people are seeking manipulative therapy from an osteopath or a chiropractor. The treatment involves the manual adjustment of the joints in the spine, and is beneficial to a wide variety of disorders, particularly spinal problems.

Medical manipulation is practised by some doctors and physiotherapists (see Chapter 7). Their techniques are not significantly different from osteopathic or chiropractic techniques, except that

medical manipulators are more likely to use traction when treating the neck. The major distinction is that doctors attempt to make a medical diagnosis before starting treatment, and then concentrate on resolving that particular problem. Non-medical manipulators often treat simply by feeling which spinal segment is at fault. They may approach the problem indirectly and continue treatment after the symptoms have disappeared. The three case histories at the end of this chapter (see pages 96 to 100) demonstrate the different techniques used in the various branches of manipulation.

OSTEOPATHY AND CHIROPRACTIC

Although osteopaths and chiropractors have increasingly tended to conform to basic medical training, most retain a holistic approach to the patient. Unconstrained by the rigours of medical scrutiny, with its emphasis on diagnosis, they view back pain in the context of disorders of the whole spine, pelvis, lower limbs, and muscle imbalance. The therapists are likely to give advice on diet – a factor which conventional doctors might not link to back pain. Qualified osteopaths and chiropractors have undergone a four year training in anatomy, physiology, biochemistry and clinical examination and treatment of musculo-skeletal disorders. They also

learn a certain amount of pathology. In the United States, osteopaths may train for seven years and are fully medically qualified. In Australia, chiropractors train for five years.

The difference between osteopathy and chiropractic is quite subtle. The chiropractor is perhaps more likely to see the problem in terms of the spine's structure, in particular the position of the bones. For this reason he tends to use X-rays more frequently than the osteopath, and his treatment is aimed at repositioning specific bones using thrusting techniques. The osteopath emphasizes function – that is, abnormal movement of the joint as the essential

MANIPULATION: A BRIEF HISTORY

Traditionally, bone setting and manipulation were skills practised by country people, quite often the shepherd or the local blacksmith, who had no medical training and simply passed down their knowledge from generation to generation. When medical schools were established in the 1850s, manipulation and massage did not form part of the curriculum, which started with dissecting a corpse rather than getting the feel of living tissue. Manipulation remained in the hands of laymen and to some extent the doctors and patients lost out. Manipulators did not always have the broader medical knowledge of doctors (though sometimes this helped them to look at their patients as people rather than focusing too narrowly on the affected part of the body). Doctors often failed to help their patients through being ignorant and indeed bigoted about this particular field, and ordinary people suffered because often they did not know who to turn to. Fortunately, the situation is now much better. More and more doctors are trained in manipulative techniques, or are referring their patients with back problems to qualified osteopaths and chiropractors.

Osteopathy was founded in America in 1874 by Andrew Taylor Still, the first school being set up in 1892. This was before the medical profession in the United States had come under the control of hospital-based physicians and surgeons. About 20 years later another American, Daniel D. Palmer, founded chiropractic. Originally both schools of thought claimed to have a comprehensive system of treatment for almost all disorders simply by manipulating the patient's spine.

feature in a spinal disorder. He tends to use leverage rather than thrusting, and often employs a rhythmic stretching of the ligaments around the joint to restore the optimal range of movement. His techniques are aimed at loosening and freeing rather than at repositioning. However, both practitioners recognize that structure and function cannot be separated, and their methods and techniques overlap. Furthermore, techniques and skills differ between individual therapists, and each practitioner develops his own method.

Consulting a practitioner

Your first appointment with an osteopath or chiropractor does not need to be arranged through your doctor. You are perfectly free to contact either practitioner directly, but it is wise to inform your doctor if you do this. If manipulation has helped you in the past, and the problem recurs, it will probably help you again.

There are, however, some conditions in which it is of no value and can even be dangerous, which is why you or your doctor must know what is wrong with you – at least in general terms – before you have manipulation. Very occasionally, back pain can be a symptom of cancer, for example, in which case manipulation is inappropriate and could be dangerous. In inflammatory conditions such as ankylosing spondylitis (see page 63), where the spinal ligaments calcify to lock the spine rigid, manipulation is of no use, though not actually dangerous. A well-qualified and conscientious manipulator will discriminate between those who will and those who will not benefit from manipulation.

Each practitioner, whether medically qualified or not, varies in his approach. Most will ask questions and examine you in much the same way as a physiotherapist (see page 82), and may include some other methods of examination according to his own preference.

CAN MANIPULATION RELIEVE PAIN?

If you are considering whether to consult a manipulator, you will probably want to know whether he can alleviate your pain. Unfortunately, it is impossible to give a definite answer. No two cases are identical – even slight differences of age, weight, fitness or will to recover can affect the success of manipulation. So, too, can the rapport between therapist and patient. Whether you are referred to a practitioner by your doctor or approach one directly, it is important that you are able to get on well with the therapist and trust him.

If you are going to benefit from this treatment, you will probably feel some relief from pain after the first two or three sessions. If the pain is unchanged by then, your condition is unlikely to improve with further sessions of manipulative treatment.

Effects on the nervous system

If muscles have weakened because a nerve has been pinched, manipulation can free the nerve, allowing strength and movement to be restored. Although the autonomic nervous system, which controls involuntary processes such as heartbeat and digestion, is not contained within the spinal canal, it links up with nerves inside it. These functions can therefore be affected by disorders of the spine, so conditions such as migraine, premenstrual tension and constipation can all be improved with manipulative treatment.

Manipulation may sometimes be used preventatively, to keep the spine mobile. Such treatment may delay degenerative changes, or, if you already have osteoarthritis, it might prevent acute problems such as dislodged facet joints.

CONDITIONS THAT MAY RESPOND

The conditions listed below and opposite are those that are most likely to respond to and benefit from treatment by a manipulative therapist.

Osteoarthritis

When this degenerative disease affects the lumbar spine, the condition may be helped by gentle manipulation. The practitioner will soon have a fairly clear idea of the limits of the help he can give; this condition cannot be cured, but some help can be given to maintain mobility. When there is inflammation of the joints, however, manipulation will not be helpful.

Disc prolapse

If you have severe lumbago, you will probably be unable to move your back without great pain, so the practitioner will have to visit you in your own home. Sometimes gentle manual traction can bring relief, but in any case the practitioner will carefully help you to find the most comfortable resting position. After a few days' rest, your pain may have subsided enough for you to have some very gentle manipulation.

Neck pain

In acute cases of wry neck, which is often caused by sleeping in an awkward position, manipulation has only a limited application. Massage can relax your taut muscles and gentle traction can begin to restore movement. However, the ligaments around the joint may be overstretched and inflamed so that any joint movement is painful. Here again the practitioner will apply traction very carefully, and then place your head and neck as close as possible to the normal resting position. He will repeat this process every ten minutes. Any more active manipulation can worsen the condition; traction and rotation are done in gradual stages to restore the normal position.

Sciatica

In sciatica, both acute and chronic, there is quite often constant pain. If a disc protrusion is causing pain in the leg without any symptoms of nerve damage, manipulation may be helpful. If there are neurological symptoms such as numbness or muscle weakness, manipulation may not help. Even so, the therapist may be able to help you find a position which relieves the pain. There are few guidelines here: sometimes you will be more comfortable standing up than lying down, and sometimes you will find that a position or movement which relieved the pain on one occasion fails on the next.

Sacroiliac strain

Some people have more mobile sacroiliac joints than others. If the elasticity of the ligaments allows a lot of movement, the ilium may rotate too far on the sacrum. When this happens, the ligaments over the joints are strained. Manipulation can align the two bones properly and ease the strain, but too much manipulation can stretch the ligaments and make the condition worse.

Facet joint malalignment

Too much twisting or bending of the spine can cause the facet joints to slip out of alignment. Manipulation can put the joints back in the correct position. You may need some help from the manipulator to find the best resting position, so that the damage can heal. Disc or facet joint problems resulting from a whiplash injury may benefit from manual traction applied by an experienced manipulator soon after the pain and stiffness started.

Rib lesions

Sometimes the head of a rib, where it is attached to a vertebra, gets out of position. The whole rib is then either "elevated", relative to the other ribs, or "depressed". Manipulation can restore the correct position.

Chronic muscular tension

If you are suffering from chronic muscular tension, manipulation of the joints will not help to relax them. However, the practitioner may stretch the muscles rhythmically. Along with this passive stretching of muscles, you must also do exercises to strengthen specific muscles. For example, when the muscles in the lower back, which bend the spine backwards, are chronically tense and shortened, the opposing muscles in the abdomen will be stretched and weakened, so you must exercise to shorten and strengthen these muscles (see page 167). The manipulator should advise you on appropriate exercises to strengthen your muscles without straining them.

Functional scoliosis

If you have scoliosis, where the spine is curved over to one side, the success of manipulation depends on a number of factors. X-rays might show vertebral wedging, in which one side of the vertebra is narrower than the other (structural scoliosis). A spine like this cannot be straightened by manipulation since it is the shape of the bones that determines the posture.

However, if the X-rays show that the shape of the vertebrae is normal, you may be leaning over to one side to minimize pain caused, perhaps, by a disc protrusion. This is known as functional scoliosis, and manipulation may help to cure the underlying cause.

If one leg is longer than the other, the pelvis may tilt and produce changes in posture. It is easy to correct the leg length simply by raising the height of one shoe. That would correct the sideways tilt of the pelvis and gradually undo the curve further up the spine. However, this might cause more aches and pains than the adapted posture.

▥ THREE APPROACHES TO BACK PAIN ▥

The differences between osteopathy, chiropractic and medical manipulation are best demonstrated by describing a typical treatment session for each method. The three case histories that follow outline consultations, including examination methods, diagnosis and treatment, for each of the three main types of manipulation. They demonstrate the benefits to be gained from manipulative treatment for both acute and chronic problems, even if the symptoms are not confined to the spine.

ACUTE LUMBAGO
This is a fairly typical case of acute lower back pain brought on by awkward twisting and stretching of the spine.

Symptoms
Mike had been experiencing an intermittent mild ache in his lower back for some time, usually after driving, but it lasted only a few hours. However, during a game of squash he felt a sudden very sharp pain in his lower back, which eased to a dull ache for the rest of the day. The next morning, the pain was piercing again and shot down his right leg. Certain movements made it worse – bending backwards and to the right were particularly painful, so Mike adopted a position slightly bent forwards and leaning to the left. This was his first attack of acute pain, and he decided to consult an osteopath.

Examination
The osteopath made a diagnosis through physical examination, asking Mike to bend his back and describe the pain this provoked. As soon as he bent slightly to the right, Mike had sharp pain in his back and down his right leg. If he bent backwards, he felt severe pain across his lower back. Bending forwards or to the left did not hurt.

Next, Mike lay on his back, and the osteopath lifted each leg. The left one could be raised to about 60° before it was painful, but raising the right leg caused the same piercing pain. Lying on his front was painful, since this arched his lower back slightly, but with cushions under his stomach, making his lower spine flat, Mike was able to lie comfortably without pain.

Diagnosis
From this examination, the osteopath diagnosed that Mike was suffering from a protruding disc. It was bulging to the right hand side and pressing against the sciatic nerve. Since Mike was comfortable lying down with his spine straight, the osteopath deduced that the disc was not fixed in its new position, but was mobile enough to return to its original position as soon as the upper part of the spine was not pressing on it. This suggested that gentle manipulation combined with manual traction would be sufficient to cure the problem.

TREATMENT BY AN OSTEOPATH

The osteopath began by treating the muscles of Mike's back, which had seized up in an attempt to protect his damaged spine. When the muscles had relaxed, the osteopath could begin to manipulate the spinal structure itself, to encourage the disc protrusion to recede.

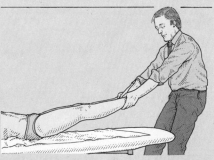

Manual traction
Mike lay on his back, holding on to the couch, and the osteopath gripped his legs and leaned back slowly to stretch Mike's spine gently. This increased the gaps between the vertebrae very slightly, in order to suck the disc protrusion back into position.

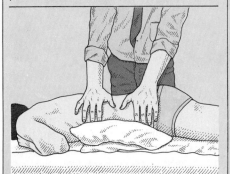

Massage
Mike lay on his front with cushions under his stomach. As well as helping to relax Mike's tense muscles, the massage stretched the spine slightly, which helped to ease the disc back into place. After about five minutes he could lie comfortably without cushions, the pain in his leg had receded, and the back pain was more central.

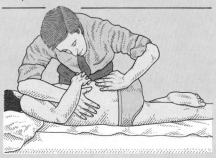

Rotational manipulation
With Mike lying on his left side, the osteopath pushed the vertebrae apart manually, by pushing the upper back away and pulling the lower back towards him, thus encouraging the protruding nucleus to return to its original position. The manipulation was repeated with Mike lying on his other side.

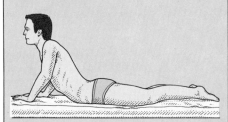

Passive extension exercise
After about 20 minutes the osteopath raised the head of the couch, arching Mike's back slightly. He asked Mike to arch his back more by pressing up with his hands under his shoulders while keeping his hips on the couch (see page 157). He repeated this four or five times. The exercise hurt slightly to begin with, but the pain decreased with each application.

RECOVERY

After this treatment, Mike no longer had pain in his leg, he could stand straight and bend backwards. The osteopath instructed him to rest for a few days and to repeat the passive extension exercise twice a day. Several days later Mike had another session of manipulation, and needed no further treatment.

WHIPLASH INJURY

This case history shows how manipulation of spinal joints can cure problems that are not always associated with disorders of the spine.

Symptoms

Jill approached a chiropractor for help with severe migraine headaches combined with nausea, vomiting and visual disturbances during the onset of these headaches. She also complained of intermittent pins and needles radiating down her right arm into her thumb and index finger.

Examination

The chiropractor began his investigation by taking a medical history. He discovered that she had been experiencing these symptoms since suffering a whiplash injury in a car accident three years earlier. She had not been X-rayed at that time, and had no other illnesses. She took pain-killers for the headaches.

Next, the chiropractor checked her blood pressure, and the reflexes of her arm muscles by tapping gently on the tendons. Then he checked that the pupils of her eyes could contract and dilate properly. Her blood pressure and eye reflexes were normal, but the reflexes in her right arm were slightly slower than those in her left arm. He rotated and extended her neck to check that the vertebral artery, which supplies blood to the brain, was not constricted, and found no abnormality.

Finally, he examined her spine for ability to twist and bend. He found that she could twist her head to the left easily and without any pain, but that her neck was stiff and painful when she tried to turn it to the right. Bending her head forwards caused pain in her mid back. The greatest stiffness was between the fifth and sixth cervical vertebrae. Jill's lower spine was examined while she lay face down on a couch. The chiropractor felt each joint individually, and discovered that her mid back was slightly stiff between the sixth and seventh thoracic vertebrae.

The chiropractor arranged for Jill to have X-rays of her spine, to discover whether there were any major joint changes, and to exclude the possibility of a serious underlying disorder. The results of the X-rays were normal.

Diagnosis

The chiropractor diagnosed that the whiplash injury had resulted in stiffness between the fifth and sixth vertebrae in Jill's neck and the sixth and seventh thoracic vertebrae. This lack of mobility, or perhaps scar tissue from the accident, interfered with the nerves in that area so that they could not function properly. This accounted for the pins and needles and the sluggish reflex in the right arm, as well as for her migraine headaches.

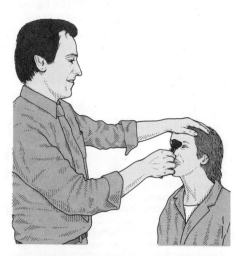

Checking the eye reflexes
The chiropractor shone a light into each of Jill's eyes to make sure that her pupils were able to react properly to the light by becoming narrower.

TREATMENT BY A CHIROPRACTOR

Chiropractors have specially designed couches divided into four sections, which can be raised or lowered independently of each other. This enables the chiropractor to use sharp thrusting movements to manipulate the spine. By lowering the appropriate section of the couch at the moment he thrusts down on a vertebra, the chiropractor can increase the movement of one segment of the back while minimizing the force on the spine. The chiropractor treated two vertebrae in Jill's back in this way, checking the mobility of her back and neck each time.

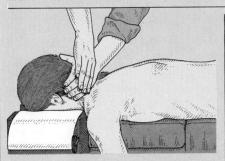

1 Jill lay face down on the couch. The upper half was raised about 5cm (2in) above the other half. The chiropractor placed his hand on the spinous process of her fifth cervical vertebra, and thrust down sharply, simultaneously lowering the raised half of the couch.

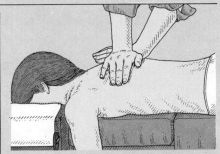

2 To treat the vertebra in Jill's mid back, the chiropractor placed the heel of one hand over the spinous process of the sixth thoracic vertebra with his other hand on top. He then thrust down in a short, sharp movement, to adjust the position of the vertebra.

RECOVERY

After this treatment, Jill stopped getting migraines, and her spine was less stiff. She needed three more sessions before she was able to flex and extend her spine fully. The nerves were no longer affected, and her symptoms disappeared.

AGEING SPINE

Manipulation is of value in general back pain, even if the joints are not out of position, as this case demonstrates.

Symptoms

A 60 year old lorry driver, John, consulted a medical manipulator about an acute attack of lower back pain. He had been stooping to pick up the tail flap of his truck when the pain started. Three days after this he was able to stand up straight, but only with difficulty, and when he changed position there was a sharp pain in his lower back on the right hand side. John had had several attacks of back pain over the last few years, and a background of general aching.

Examination

The doctor took a detailed case history. He discovered that John had been experiencing some bowel disturbance, including the passing of some blood and mucus, and was having to pass small amounts of urine very frequently. He was also caring for an invalid wife.

The doctor performed a thorough physical examination. He asked John to bend forwards, backwards and to each side, in order to check the flexibility of his spine. He found that John's movement was restricted in two directions and that his back ached when he tried to bend too far. Then, with John lying on his front, the doctor felt each spinal segment individually. John's spine was particularly sensitive to pressure between the fourth and fifth lumbar vertebrae. The doctor's investigation also included a rectal examination, to assess the size and shape of his prostate gland, and to discover whether there was a tumour in the rectum.

The doctor arranged for blood tests and X-rays of the spine, to find out whether an underlying disease could account for John's symptoms. The blood tests were normal, and the X-rays revealed no more than the usual wear and tear for a spine of that age.

Diagnosis

The doctor suspected that John had a minor disc protrusion, bulging to the right, between the fourth and fifth lumbar vertebrae, and that the facet joints and ligaments in his lower back were worn and causing instability. John had the symptoms of osteoarthritis, and changes due to degeneration were visible on the X-rays.

TREATMENT BY A MEDICAL MANIPULATOR

The doctor rotated John's spine carefully using a rotation with distraction technique — in other words, rotating the spine while simultaneously easing the joints open on one side. He then asked John to stand up and checked his movements again. Only bending forwards was painful this time. The doctor then applied a second manipulation with John lying face down, and again checked his ability to move.

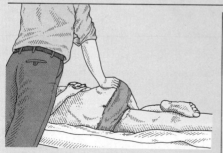

1 The doctor placed one hand on John's right shoulder and the other on John's right hip. While pushing his shoulder and hip down to rotate John's spine, the doctor leaned forwards, so that his body weight pushed his arms apart, thus stretching John's right side and slightly distracting the spinal joints on that side.

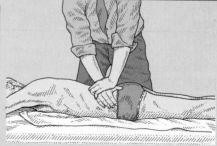

2 John lay face down and the doctor placed the heel of one hand on the left (painless) side between the fourth and fifth lumbar vertebrae. He then leaned over to apply a sudden downwards force angled towards the midline.

RECOVERY

After two treatments, John had a full range of movement and the doctor advised him on posture and lifting techniques in caring for his wife. He was also offered ligament sclerosant therapy (see page 104) in order to stabilize the affected lumbar segments.

9
Drugs and injections

Whatever the cause of your back pain, a doctor is very likely to treat it with drugs. Recently, drugs have received a lot of adverse publicity, and doctors who use standard pharmacological treatments have been contrasted with homeopaths and herbalists who, it is claimed, take a more holistic approach.

Nevertheless, a doctor who does prescribe drugs to help you recover from your back pain may well be acting on sound holistic principles. It is perfectly possible, for example, that muscle relaxants and pain-killers, combined with bed rest, are the best way of putting you into the optimum mental and physical state for the healing process to start. However, your doctor may not have considered other approaches, which are often more effective than drugs.

TREATMENT WITH DRUGS

Doctors use a wide range of drugs to relieve and cure back pain. These range from simple pain-killers available over the counter which may help you to get over an acute attack, to drugs for specific conditions, such as chymopapain, used to shrink protruding discs.

Simple pain-killers
Pain-killers such as codeine, aspirin and panadol are available over the counter in most parts of the world and are useful for coping with mild to moderate pain.

Combination drugs
Paracetamol, or aspirin or codeine combined with another drug, can relieve mild to moderate pain. These combination drugs are available over the counter from chemists in many countries throughout the world.

Strong analgesics (pain-killers)
These include narcotics such as morphine and pethidine, and non-narcotics such as meptazinol and buprenorphine. If you are in severe pain, unable to find comfort in any position and unable to sleep, you should be given a strong pain-killer, particularly if your pain continues for more than 12 to 24 hours.

Non-narcotics have few side-effects, but narcotics may cause constipation and drowsiness. Unfortunately, though non-narcotics are often less effective than narcotics, many doctors are rather reluctant to prescribe strong narcotic analgesics because they are afraid that the patient may become addicted. In short-term acute pain this is an unnecessary fear, and even long-term use is unlikely to result in dependency among people in severe pain who are in genuine need of strong pain-killers. But recent evidence suggests that some people are naturally prone to addiction, and your doctor should be aware of this risk. If you are worried about this, discuss it with your doctor.

If you are suffering from severe sciatica or brachialgia caused by nerve root compression, it is my belief that good pain relief in the early stages will help to prevent the sort of emotional reaction to pain which can delay recovery.

Muscle relaxants

In acute neck pain or lumbago, when the muscles tend to tighten up to protect the painful area from further injury, these drugs can be useful. If you are highly strung or apprehensive, your muscles may stay tense for longer than necessary after injury and can remain fixed like this even after the injury has started to heal. Massage or relaxation therapy may help (see pages 171 to 173), but if these are not available, you may be given diazepam or a similar drug for two or three days.

The drawback to this is that it will slow you down mentally and make you drowsy, and long-term use can lead to dependency. Unfortunately, muscle relaxants are all too often prescribed for people who have no real need for them.

Anti-inflammatory drugs

Many doctors now prescribe these routinely for all musculo-skeletal pain to ensure that joints do not become inflamed. However, they are really effective only for treating inflammatory

disorders such as ankylosing spondylitis (see page 63). It is debatable whether they are beneficial for non-inflammatory conditions. These drugs can produce side-effects of drowsiness, skin rashes, nausea, gastric irritation, diarrhoea and unfortunately the occasional internal haemorrhage. Other side-effects which can occur are due to allergy or fluid retention. There are over 50 varieties of this type of drug, and although the newest ones produce fewer side-effects, they still do not offer better relief from pain and stiffness than standard drugs such as codeine.

Steroids

These are synthetic drugs which are very similar to the body's natural steroid hormones. They are prescribed in much larger quantities than the body is used to, and they work by a powerful anti-inflammatory action.

Some conditions which affect all the joints of the body, including the spine, can be helped with corticosteroids. In its later stages, rheumatoid arthritis, for example, can affect the spine and is sometimes treated effectively with steroids taken by mouth.

There has been a lot of negative comment about cortisone and steroids in recent years, because long-term oral steroids have side-effects such as weight gain, acne, hirsutism (hairiness), high blood pressure, diabetes, reduced resistance to infection and osteoporosis (see page 58).

It is, however, quite a different matter to be given a much smaller quantity of corticosteroid in a local injection to reduce swelling and irritation around a nerve root or to treat inflammation in a joint. This treatment should relieve your symptoms, and because it is administered directly to the affected area, you will probably have no side-effects whatsoever, so do not let bad publicity about steroids in general put you off.

Drugs for osteoporosis

If your bones have degenerated severely and become thin and brittle, some mineral and vitamin supplements can help strengthen them or slow down the rate of degeneration. Calcium and vitamin D may build up the bones again, and a new drug called Ossopan is extremely effective.

INJECTIONS

If your doctor suggests that you have any of the following treatments, do not be alarmed at the prospect of a course of injections. The treatment will be administered by an experienced and well-trained specialist and any pain caused by an injection will probably be minimal compared with your previous pain.

Injections are a marvellously accurate and effective way of delivering treatment to the specific source of trouble. Why take a general, non-specific course of treatment when a local, specific treatment, without risk of any side-effects, can be given?

However, you should not expect immediate relief from your symptoms: it may take several sessions before your back pain begins to recede. The success of the treatment also depends to some extent on you following your doctor's advice on how to look after your back both between sessions and after the course of treatment has finished.

MUSCULAR INJECTIONS

Trigger points (see page 49) are often treated successfully with a course of local injections containing a small dose of corticosteroid combined with local anaesthetic, unless the joints nearby are the source of the problem. If this is the case, the joints themselves have to be treated first, and the muscles should then relax of their own accord. Local injections are often most helpful if they are combined with stretching exercises and a cooling spray to help muscles relax. The treatment can be given in your doctor's surgery.

LIGAMENT INJECTIONS

If your pain comes from sprained ligaments, you might find that the injury is slow to heal. A few people need a local injection of steroid with some local anaesthetic added.

Procedure

The doctor will identify your strained ligament with his fingers and inject a drop at one end, shift the needle slightly and inject another drop, working this way until the ligament has been injected along its entire length and breadth.

You may feel some soreness or aching for 24 to 48 hours after a steroid injection. Your doctor will tell you to rest the joint by refraining from excessive lifting, carrying and bending. You will also be advised not to sit in one position for long periods. After about ten days your doctor will see you again so that he can assess your progress.

The reason why you need to rest is because the collagen (protein fibre) that provides tension in the ligaments is affected for the first ten to 14 days after a steroid injection, which makes the tissues a bit weaker. After this the ligament collagen returns to normal. A small amount of steroid will probably be absorbed into your blood, but not enough to cause any side-effects.

SCLEROSANT THERAPY

Chronic ligament strain, particularly in the lower back and sacroiliac joints, is common in people whose backs have become unstable due, for example, to narrow discs causing the facet joints to cram together, or perhaps to a recurrent dislodgement of the sacroiliac joint. The treatment for this is ligament sclerosant therapy, known as prolotherapy in the United States.

Normal mobility can be restored by injecting sclerosant into the ligaments which control the motion of the relevant segment or joint. This treatment is also helpful in mild spondylolisthesis, when one vertebra shifts slightly. Tighter ligaments help to hold the vertebra more securely in position.

Sclerosant injections contain a small amount of fibrous tissue irritant in an inert solution such as glycerine. The sclerosant stimulates the production of fibrous tissue and new collagen, and after several injections at weekly intervals the ligament will become thicker, shorter and even stronger at the junction between ligament and bone.

In the United States you are most likely to receive this treatment from a medically trained osteopath, while in Britain it is almost exclusively given by orthopaedic physicians, for the most part practising privately.

Procedure

If your lower back is the area to be treated, you will be asked to lie on your front over a pillow or cushion so that your lower back is slightly rounded. The specialist will then draw various landmarks on your back with a felt tip pen, to help him identify where the ligaments are attached.

LIGAMENT SCLEROSANT THERAPY

The doctor will be able to identify the position of the ligaments by feeling your back. He will locate the top of your hip bone on each side, and the spinous processes of your lumbar vertebrae. He will then draw a grid on your back using these bones as reference points to help him position the needle in exactly the right place. Even if the doctor wants to inject several ligaments, he will penetrate the skin at just a single point, and reposition the point of the needle under the skin to reach the ligaments.

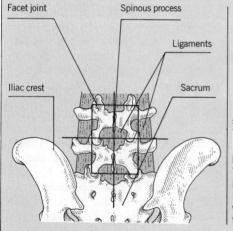

Facet joint Spinous process

Ligaments

Iliac crest Sacrum

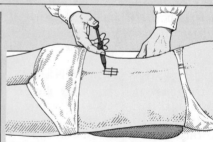

Position of the grid
The three lines across the back are half way between the spinous processes. The middle line down the back is over the centre of the vertebrae, and the lines to either side are over the facet joints.

The sclerosant solution is mixed with a local anaesthetic to dull the initial burning pain. The specialist will inject half a millilitre at either end of each ligament, and although he may wish to inject six, eight or ten ligaments in the area he will penetrate the skin at only one point.

The whole procedure can be rather painful but takes only ten to 15 minutes. If you are particularly nervous about injections, you may be given a mixture of nitrous oxide gas and air through a mask to help you relax, and some practitioners prefer you to be under a general anaesthetic. If you have not been given an anaesthetic, you will be capable of getting up and leaving the surgery.

When the local anaesthetic has worn off after two or three hours, there is a sensation of bruising. This may last for two or three days and is due to your ligaments reacting to the fibrous tissue irritant. With a skilled practitioner, there are rarely any other side-effects.

Most physicians use a course of three weekly injection treatments. You will be advised not to do too much bending or lifting during the following three weeks or so. In the fourth and fifth weeks after the treatment you should walk five kilometres (three miles) a day, to encourage local blood flow, and to strengthen and settle renewed ligaments: this is just like running in your new car or reconditioned engine. Five weeks after the last injection the doctor will examine you once more and should find that you are free of back trouble.

Results

It is important to realize that you should not expect relief from your back pain until eight weeks after the first injection is given. This is because it takes time for the new ligament tissue to grow. Some people, however, experience partial relief much sooner than this. The more important question is whether you will be free from back pain in the long term. Some people have excellent results for eight years or more, whereas others do not respond so well. It is difficult for doctors to predict how effective the treatment will be in any particular case. It is certainly worth trying, and there is no harm in repeating a course of treatment after the benefits of the first course have worn off.

EPIDURAL INJECTIONS

Injections into the epidural space can help disc protrusions causing sciatica and backache that has not responded to bed rest, pain-killers, manipulation, and other physiotherapy, including traction, exercise and massage.

If you have severe sciatica and your doctor finds symptoms of a damaged nerve root – numbness of the skin, weakness of certain muscles and absence of tendon reflex – you may benefit from an epidural.

The injection is called an "epidural" because it enters the space between the outer lining of the dura (see page 22) and the bony walls of the spinal canal. It differs from the epidural given to relieve pain in childbirth in two main ways: to treat back pain, most orthopaedic physicians inject the base of the sacrum (childbirth epidurals are given via the lower back); secondly, they use a weaker solution of local anaesthetic and add some steroid. The anaesthetic serves to numb the lining of the spinal cord, which is under pressure – usually from a protruding disc or a fragment of disc cartilage. The steroid helps to reduce the inflammation and bruising of the dural sheath which has been caused by pressure and friction.

The injection will relieve pain and allow you to return to normal activities, but it will not help the disc protrusion back into place. In most cases though, the protrusion will wither away gradually by itself, until it stops pressing on the nerve. A tiny minority of people with back pain have a loose fragment of disc cartilage, spinal stenosis or a bone pressing on a nerve. These people will not experience lasting benefit from this treatment, and will need further tests and perhaps surgery.

Procedure

The procedure is very simple, and can be carried out in the specialist's surgery. You will be asked to lie on your front over a pillow while he delivers the injection slowly over a ten-minute period. Usually the injection causes no more than a feeling of pressure in the base of the spine or the back of the legs, but sometimes it reproduces the sciatic pain at its most severe. As soon as the doctor has finished administering the injection, all pain ceases.

You will be asked to rest for ten minutes on your front followed by ten minutes on your back and the doctor may then test how high your leg can be raised while you hold it straight. You should be able to raise your leg almost vertically with no more than a shadow of the original pain. You can then get up and walk or drive home with no after effects. You will have to go back in a week or ten days so that the doctor can assess your progress.

Results

The pain may disappear and never return; it may go for a few hours, then return for a few days but fade away by the end of the week, or it may diminish gradually over the next seven days. If the injection has produced only partial relief after a week, second or third epidurals may be given at weekly intervals.

If the epidural has not worked at all, this may be because the disc protrusion is pressing too tightly against the nerve root to allow the fluid to pass between the protrusion and the dural membrane, or because the diagnosis was wrong in the first place.

EPIDURAL INJECTION

By feeling for the bones of the sacrum, the therapist will identify the base of the sacrum before administering the injection. He may have an assistant who will pull the buttocks gently apart so that the therapist can place the needle correctly. The anaesthetic and steroid solution is then injected slowly over a period of about ten minutes.

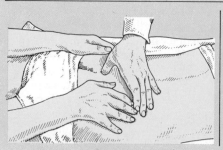

The needle enters the spinal canal through the base of the sacrum, and the anaesthetic mixed

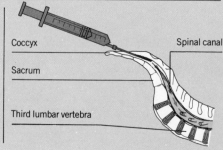

Coccyx

Sacrum

Third lumbar vertebra

Spinal canal

with steroid penetrates up the canal to reach the level of the third lumbar vertebra.

Between 40 and 70 per cent of patients obtain some relief from these injections. Complications are rare and there is no danger of making your condition worse by numbing the pain in this way. There is a slight risk that you may absorb some of the anaesthetic fluid, which will cause a temporary numbness and paralysis of the lower legs, but this will clear up in a few hours. Epidural injections do not need to be given under a general anaesthetic, and having a general anaesthetic only increases the overall risk of developing complications.

I would recommend an epidural for almost all patients who have backache or sciatica which is due to a straightforward physical cause and which has not responded to rest, manipulation or traction. The temporary discomfort of the injection itself is infinitely preferable to the unpleasant options which may be offered in its place: six weeks in a plaster jacket, prolonged traction in bed, or myelography (see page 78) and surgery (see Chapter 10).

NERVE BLOCKS

An epidural may fail to relieve pain if a nerve is trapped in the lateral canal. This can cause pain in your arm or leg without any backache (brachialgia or sciatica), and an injection of local anaesthetic and steroid to the nerve root will anaesthetize the nerve and reduce any inflammation. One or two small nerves convey pain messages to and from the facet joints and the dural sheath, and these can also be blocked and anaesthetized by this technique.

These injections are performed by a relatively small number of orthopaedic physicians who have a special interest in relieving pain from spinal disorders. They are extremely useful for chronic sufferers, and if your own doctor cannot help, he might still be able to refer you

to someone with the expertise to give these injections.

Procedure

The injection can be given in the doctor's surgery or in an out-patients' department, and there is no need for a general anaesthetic. You will be asked to lie on your front on a couch while the physician injects a small amount of local anaesthetic. The treatment is not painful, and takes about 20 to 30 minutes.

If you can stand without feeling pain after you have had the injection, or if you can raise your legs without bending them, the same place is usually injected with two millilitres of steroid suspension a few days later.

The only risk from this injection is that very occasionally the doctor may pierce the dural membrane. He will immediately recognize that he has gone too far and withdraw the needle. Although it will not be very painful, you

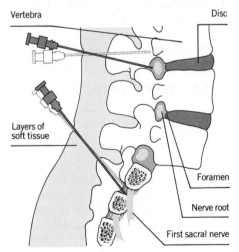

Nerve block
The tip of the needle is positioned in the foramen (the gap between two vertebrae), where a nerve emerges from the spinal canal. The anaesthetic and steroid mixture bathes the nerve root to relieve pain and reduce inflammation.

will have to lie flat for 24 hours if this happens, in order to avoid a headache or dizziness caused by any excessive leak of the cerebrospinal fluid. This is by no means as serious as it may sound. After two days the doctor will attempt the correct placement of the needle once again. Because of this albeit small risk, it is advisable to take someone with you to drive you home should you need to spend a day in bed, though if all goes as it should, you will be able to walk or drive yourself.

Results

If the relevant nerve root has been located successfully, the anaesthetic will provide several days' pain relief. When the injection is repeated with two milli-litres of steroid, prolonged or even per-manent relief may be obtained. Once again, the results are variable and it is difficult for doctors to predict how well a particular individual will respond. There are no side-effects from this in-jection. If the needle has pierced the dura, there will be no further symptoms or problems after the initial day or two's headache and dizziness.

FACET JOINT INJECTIONS

Most backache related to facet joints can be treated successfully with a combin-ation of exercise and improved posture, but if your symptoms are very severe, you may need an injection. In this case, your doctor will inject a mixture of local anaesthetic and steroid into your dam-aged facet joints. The treatment is given in the doctor's surgery, and it may be slightly painful.

Results

Unfortunately these injections do not usually provide relief for more than a few months to people suffering from osteoarthritis. If you are suffering from this degenerative disease, you may find that one of the newer techniques offered by some orthopaedic surgeons is more beneficial to you. These include rhizoly-sis, in which the nerves supplying the joint are cut, and cryocautery, in which the nerve endings in the joint capsule are freeze-burned to deaden them. They are not major operations and you will not need to stay in hospital.

Even these techniques may not pro-vide lasting relief if you have instability resulting from an operation. In this case further surgery or long-term use of anti-inflammatory drugs may be necessary.

CHEMONUCLEOLYSIS

This is a relatively new treatment for sciatica related to disc problems. It has been researched for many years and has recently been receiving much publicity as a viable alternative to surgery. The term means chemical breakdown of the nucleus of the disc.

Chymopapain, a protein-digesting enzyme derived from the papaya fruit, is purified into a concentrated solution. When a minute amount is injected into the centre of the disc, the disc material starts to break down, so that the pro-truded pulp is under less pressure. In a few weeks the disc shrinks and your sciatica will be relieved. The technique is becoming more and more popular among orthopaedic surgeons.

Procedure

You will be admitted to hospital for two or three days for this treatment. The injection is given in the operating theatre or radiology department under X-ray control. There is no need for you to have a general anaesthetic, but you may well have a "pre-med", or sedative, injection to help you to relax for the procedure. The specialist will identify which disc needs treatment, either by myelogram (see page 78) or sometimes by discogram (see page 80), and then inject the powerful fruit-juice extract, with you lying either on your front or on your side. X-ray focusing tubes will be beamed at you from two angles so that the operator can check that his needle is in the centre of the relevant disc.

Soon after the injection you may experience quite severe pain, and for the first few days following the injection you might need a pain-killer.

Results

Between 50 and 80 per cent of patients benefit from this treatment, but there can be some complications. These include neurological complications and severe allergic reaction, so if you are allergic to meat tenderizer, melon or papaya, you will not be able to receive this treatment.

Recent studies in Europe and Great Britain show that the risk of complications has been reduced and is now less than in surgery. Once a disc has been injected and shrunken in this way, the physical effect is permanent. Therefore if the correct disc has been treated, the pain relief should also be permanent. If, however, the treatment fails to relieve the pain caused by pressure on the nerve root, then surgery will probably be recommended to you.

DRUGS FOR BACK PAIN

Type of drug	Action	Example
Simple pain-killers	for relief of mild to moderate pain, act locally and centrally (via the brain)	aspirin, codeine, paracetamol
Combination drugs	for relief of mild to moderate pain	aspirin, codeine or paracetamol combined with dextropoxyphene or meprobamate
Stronger pain-killers	for relief of moderate to severe pain	dihydro-codeine tartrate
Non-narcotic strong analgesics	for relief of severe pain	meptazinol, buprenorphine
Narcotic analgesics	for relief of severe pain (act via the brain)	pethidine, morphine, pentazocine
Muscle relaxants	provide relief by central (brain) sedation and peripheral (muscular) relaxation	diazepam
Non-steroidal anti-inflammatory drugs	reduce pain by inhibiting enzymes at the site of injury or inflammation	ibuprofen, naproxen, indomethacin
Drugs to break down protein and collagen	break down protein and collagen, causing disc to shrink	chymopapain
Steroids (Cortisone type agents)	suppress inflammation	triamcinolone acetonide triamcinolone hexacetonide
Anti-depressants	counteract the psychological effects of chronic pain	amitryptyline
Anabolic steroids	break down scar tissue (still in experimental stage)	stanazolol

10
Surgery

Only a tiny minority of people with back problems need surgery, and if your doctor suggests an operation you will probably have already tried several other treatments unsuccessfully. Surgery is the only way to deal with certain kinds of infections and tumours, and in these cases it may be life-saving. If your spine is structurally damaged and other treatment has failed, you will need some specialized investigations (described in Chapter 6) to discover whether your condition could be cured with an operation. The most common reason for spinal surgery is to treat disc problems. In Britain alone, over 6,000 operations are performed each year for disc prolapses. A small proportion of surgery is done to stabilize fractures or other segments of the spine where nerves are being compressed and damaged.

The benefits and risks

Surgery to the spine now has a very high success rate regardless of the patient's age, owing to increasingly accurate diagnosis as much as to improved surgical techniques. The risks from spinal operations include those involved in all surgery: reaction to the anaesthetic, chest infection, blood clots, haemorrhage and infection of the wound. Although these complications are sometimes serious, they are extremely rare these days. In addition to these, there is a slim chance of damage to the spinal

cord. Approximately one in every 5,000 operations results in nerve damage leading to paralysis, and about one in 50 patients suffer from mild, temporary complications, such as bladder infections. The mortality rate is low, about 0.3 per cent, usually caused by severe damage to the spinal cord or to a blood clot becoming lodged in the lungs.

If you have any fears about having an operation, it is important to discuss them with your doctor or specialist. He will probably be able to relieve your anxieties and make you confident that surgery will improve your condition.

Most sciatica patients are still free from severe pain ten years after surgery, and only between five and 15 per cent need further surgery. The vast majority of patients benefit, but some problems are not cured completely by surgery, and it is important to have realistic expectations. Roughly a quarter of patients undergoing discectomy or laminectomy (see opposite and page 113) experience residual back pain or discomfort, though this is minimal compared with the level of pain experienced before surgery.

Operable conditions

The most common spinal operations are undertaken to relieve lower back pain and sciatica. They are all done under general anaesthetic. Conditions which may be treated surgically include disc prolapse (usually if it causes sciatica), central or lateral canal stenosis, severe instability in the lower back, severe facet joint disease and severe spondylolisthesis. You will probably be offered surgery only after other treatment has failed, but in some circumstances it is best to operate immediately to avoid damage to the spinal cord. These include the following conditions:

● A large disc prolapse causing pressure on the spinal cord, which would give you severe back pain, severe sciatic pain in one or both legs, marked loss of sensation and weak muscles in the lower limbs, and bladder and bowel weakness or incontinence. This is rare but happens when most of the central, pulpy part of the disc bulges into the spinal canal. All doctors and specialists are alerted to the possibility of this happening, and you would be unwise not to follow their advice for urgent surgery.

● Occasionally this kind of prolapsed disc may cause only deep pain in the region of the sacrum or coccyx, pain in the crutch and groin areas, and some symptoms of bladder weakness or incontinence. You may not experience leg pain, muscle weakness and loss of sensation. If your symptoms do not disappear quickly with rest in a hospital bed, you may need a myelogram and surgery.

● Sometimes there is back and/or leg pain of some weeks' duration which after a while causes progressive signs of damage to the nerves. Provided your doctor or specialist is examining you regularly to check the degree of muscle weakness and loss of sensation, this should not be missed.

● Sometimes tumours of the vertebrae or infections in the disc space and around the spinal column can produce similar symptoms. These would need urgent surgery or antibiotic medicines.

DISCECTOMY

This operation is used in a few cases of **disc prolapse**, when the protrusion does not return to its original position, and has to be removed surgically. In a discectomy, most of the disc is left in place, while the protruding piece is removed. If your doctor suggests this operation, he will refer you to a specialist who will assess your condition, probably using sophisticated X-ray techniques including myelography, electromyography or a CT scan (see Chapter 6). These will inform the specialist whether you could benefit from a discectomy. If he is at all uncertain about the diagnosis, the surgeon will not perform the operation.

Procedure
The surgeon makes a cut through the skin and muscles to the ligaments which lie across the back of the spinal canal, then carefully cuts through these to expose the nerves. These are gently drawn aside to reveal the protruding disc. The protruding part of the disc and any loose fragments of cartilage are removed, and the surgeon will then check the width of the lateral canal to ensure that the nerve root it contains is under no pressure. If the canal is too narrow, he may remove tiny fragments of bone to widen it (see decompression operation, page 112). The layers are then stitched carefully back together, and the operation is complete.

Some surgeons are trained in microscopic surgery, and perform this operation through a very small incision not much more than 2cm (1in) long, with the aid of a binocular microscope.

Discectomy

The main body of the disc is left untouched, but the surgeon removes the part that is protruding and causing pain.

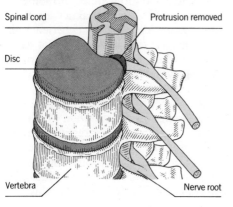

Spinal cord — Protrusion removed

Disc

Vertebra — Nerve root

Recuperation

You will be surprised at the dramatic relief from pain in your leg if this operation has been successful. The pain from the operative wound is often mild in contrast to the sciatic pain which you have been experiencing over the previous weeks. Within two to three days the nurses will encourage you to stand up and walk around, but they will advise against sitting or bending for the first week, since this may stretch the wound. In order to prevent scar tissue forming around the nerve root, you should practise straight leg raises several times a day starting on the third day after the operation: lie on your back and slowly raise the leg that used to be painful, keeping it straight.

After you have been moving around for a week or so, your stitches or sutures will be removed, and you will be allowed to go home. You will not be able to do any heavy lifting or carrying, and surgeons will recommend wearing a light corset to support your back for the first few weeks. Most people are able to return to light duties around the house and to office or sedentary work within about two months of this operation. You should avoid any heavy manual work for at least three months. Some specialists would advise you against returning to heavy manual work ever again, but if you are young and previously fit, provided that you use proper lifting and handling techniques, you should be able to return to your work. Discectomy causes remarkably little upset to the system in general and people readily return to a normal life.

A disc generally does not become herniated or prolapsed, however, unless it has become weakened by recurrent injury. This implies that some extra care throughout life is necessary: avoid becoming overweight, do daily exercises (see Chapter 14) and follow the advice given in Chapter 13.

Eight or nine out of every ten people who have a discectomy obtain complete relief from pain in the leg; between a quarter to one half of them still experience some backache. This is probably due to minor instability in the lower back which existed before the prolapse.

DECOMPRESSION

If your spinal canal is too narrow at one point (**central** or **lateral canal stenosis**), it might need to be widened surgically to relieve pressure on nerves. The canal may be narrow due to a disc protruding into it, which is cured by a

discectomy; however it may be narrowed by bony spurs (see Osteophytes, page 59) growing on the vertebrae, or you might have been born with a narrow spinal canal. Sometimes when a vertebra shifts in **spondylolisthesis**, it

Decompression

Tiny chips of bone are removed to reduce pressure on the nerves. There are two main types of decompression operation. In a laminectomy, bone is removed from the lamina; in a facetectomy, part of the inner edge of the facet joint is removed.

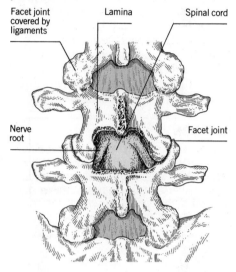

Facet joint covered by ligaments | Lamina | Spinal cord

Nerve root | Facet joint

can press on nerves in the central canal. In all these cases, small pieces of bone have to be chipped away in order to leave enough room for the spinal cord. These

conditions can be diagnosed by the specialized X-rays and scans described in Chapter 6, but sometimes a surgeon discovers the problem only during a discectomy while doing his routine check on the width of the lateral canal.

Procedure

The surgeon makes an incision to expose the bone, and removes minute amounts of bone from the vertebra. If your spinal canal is too narrow at more than one level, this operation can be extended either up or down without making any other incision.

The surgeon may check to see if the blood circulation to your dural sheath is impaired because of pressure within the spinal canal. If this has happened, he will extend the decompression operation upwards to restore circulation.

Recuperation

You will be able to get up and walk about two or three days after the operation. After seven to ten days you will be allowed home, but will be instructed to avoid strenuous exercise and lifting for about three months.

SPINAL FUSION

If X-rays show that a segment of your lower spine moves too much when you bend over (**lumbar instability**), you may be advised to have a fusion operation. Excessive movement of any part of the spine can cause back pain or intermittent sciatica. The fusion operation will cure these symptoms, but since it leaves one section of the back rigid, doctors are reluctant to consider the operation unless other treatment has been unsuccessful.

A fusion operation may also be recommended if you have **severe facet joint disease**, which might make the joints slip out of alignment frequently. This frequently happens when the spine degenerates with age, or if you have had a serious disc prolapse which has put extra strain on the facet joints.

Spondylolisthesis, when a vertebra slips out of alignment, can be treated with a fusion operation regardless of whether the problem is caused by a fracture or by degenerative changes. The operation will probably be recommended to adolescents who have severe spondylolisthesis which is damaging nerves, and causing pain, tingling or numbness in the legs. Adults who have degenerative spondylolisthesis may need a fusion operation, but if the only symptom is leg pain, without any accompanying back pain, you could be treated with a decompression operation.

Recuperation

This type of operation is more traumatic than a simple discectomy. You will be kept in bed for two to three weeks and then perhaps allowed up with a corset.

Your surgeon might prefer you to use a full plaster cast for six to eight weeks before you are allowed to move your spine freely. The main aim of this after-care is to allow the fusion to become solid. It takes anything from six months to one year to achieve the full effects of a fusion operation, so you should not look for immediate relief of symptoms.

In the past, a fusion operation was often performed at the same time as a standard discectomy to treat a prolapsed disc, in order to prevent further disc

FUSION OPERATION

There are two main methods of fusion, though there are many variations on each one. Both involve taking small pieces of bone from some other part of the body (normally the pelvis), and using them as a graft between two vertebrae. Sometimes several segments of the lower back are unstable and are fused by one of these techniques. The spine is usually approached from the back, but occasionally it is reached through an incision in the side or the front of the abdomen.

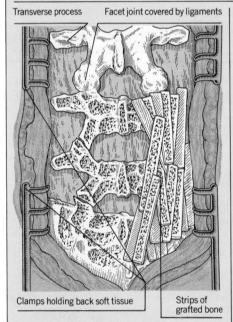

Transverse process   Facet joint covered by ligaments

Clamps holding back soft tissue | Strips of grafted bone

Posterolateral fusion
Strips of bone are placed over the facet joints, between the transverse processes, either on just one side of the vertebra, or on both sides.

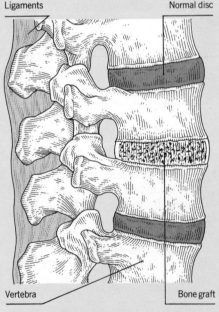

Ligaments   Normal disc

Vertebra | Bone graft

Posterior interbody fusion
The entire disc is removed and bits of bone are put in the disc space between the vertebrae to fuse the two vertebrae together.

herniation or backache. It is now recognized, though, that this combination is no more successful than simply removing the prolapse.

A fusion operation is chosen by some surgeons if, following back surgery such as decompression or discectomy, the patient still complains of low back pain. If there was no clear diagnosis of instability in the first place, only a small percentage of fusion operations are successful. Some surgeons even try more spinal fusion if the first operation has failed, but this is rarely beneficial.

SURGERY FOR SCOLIOSIS

In most cases of scoliosis (a sideways curve of the spine), the curve is very slight, and may cause no pain whatsoever. However, very severe structural scoliosis can produce considerable deformity, and you may need surgery to straighten your spine. The operation is most commonly done in early adolescence, since this is when the most severe spinal curvatures develop.

Procedure

The most common form of surgical treatment for scoliosis is the insertion of a Harrington rod. This is a telescopic metal rod which is wedged alongside the vertebrae on the concave side of the curve. During the operation, the rod is elongated to open the curve, and then the entire curved section is fused with chips of bone taken from the hip bone. If the scoliosis is very severe, you may need a compression Harrington rod on the other side of the curve.

In another method, the spine is approached from the front, and the discs between the vertebrae forming the curve are removed. Bolts are drilled transversely through the vertebrae and then crimped onto a steel cable lying

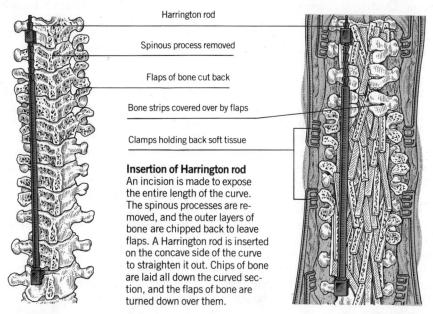

Harrington rod

Spinous process removed

Flaps of bone cut back

Bone strips covered over by flaps

Clamps holding back soft tissue

Insertion of Harrington rod
An incision is made to expose the entire length of the curve. The spinous processes are removed, and the outer layers of bone are chipped back to leave flaps. A Harrington rod is inserted on the concave side of the curve to straighten it out. Chips of bone are laid all down the curved section, and the flaps of bone are turned down over them.

115

down the convex side. The whole assembly is then tightened, thus pulling the spine straight.

Recuperation

If you have either of these operations, you will be in hospital for about two and a half weeks, and off school or work for a month. You will have to avoid sport for between six months and a year.

The operation will result in a very stiff back. In most cases, the operation will leave the ribs slightly prominent on one side. If this is particularly deforming, you can have cosmetic surgery to reduce the prominence.

SURGERY FOR COCCYDINIA

If pain resulting from a fall on the coccyx has not cleared up after several months, surgery is sometimes necessary. This involves removing the last two or three segments of the coccyx. If there has been a fracture, it is possible that it has not reunited and the loose fragment can be removed, giving relief from pain.

Recuperation

The operation is relatively minor and you can be up and walking about in a few days. Obviously, you will not be able to sit up until the wound from the operation is healed, but you can be back at work in most occupations within two to three weeks.

SURGERY OF THE NECK

The problems that occur in the neck are much the same as those in the lower spine. Doctors are more reluctant to recommend surgery, though, since any damage to the spinal cord in the neck could be fatal or result in all four limbs becoming paralysed. However, in some conditions there is a risk of the spinal cord becoming damaged through compression of the nerves, so you might need an urgent operation. These conditions include a disc protruding into the central canal, dislodged bones or bony spurs pressing on nerves, or a large tumour.

FUSION OPERATION

If a **disc prolapse** in your neck does not recover after nine months or a year of treatment, you may need surgery. Nerves in the neck can be compressed by spurs growing on the vertebrae (**cervical spondylosis**). This may damage

your spinal cord, particularly if segments in your neck are too mobile. The degree of mobility in your neck can be assessed by a specialized X-ray to find out whether a fusion operation could improve your condition.

Procedure

This operation will probably be done by a neurosurgeon who will remove the entire disc through an incision in the front of the neck. Most surgeons perform this operation under microscope.

Because discs in the neck are much smaller than those in the lower back, a much smaller space is left between the vertebrae once the disc is removed. The bones fuse naturally after this operation, and a bone graft is unnecessary.

Recuperation

This operation has a very high success rate. Almost 100 per cent of patients with a cervical disc prolapse are relieved of pain, and about 90 per cent of those with spondylosis benefit. You will need to be in hospital for only three or four days, but you will have to wear a soft collar for about two months. If you have a sedentary job, you should be able to return to work within a week or two, but you should not return to work which involves heavy lifting and carrying for two months or so, to allow the vertebrae to fuse completely.

FRACTURE DISLOCATION

A vertebra in the neck can sometimes become displaced after a fracture. If it does not slip back into place immediately, you will need traction to the skull to prevent damage to your spinal cord. Once the displacement has reduced, an operation will be performed either to fuse the damaged segments with bone grafts, or to fix them with wire. You will need to wear a neck brace for at least three months.

FAILURE OF SURGERY

If there is no improvement immediately after your operation, there are several possible reasons why the surgery has been unsuccessful.
- The wrong diagnosis was made, and the real cause of your pain is a tumour, spondylolisthesis or some inflammatory condition such as ankylosing spondylitis (see page 63).
- The symptoms are mainly of psychological origin.
- The operation was carried out at the wrong level.
- In an operation for a disc prolapse, there may be a second prolapsed disc at another level, or a fragment of the disc might still be lodged in the lateral canal.

If there was temporary relief, but your symptoms return, there are several possible explanations.
- The area that was operated on may have become infected.
- A cyst may have developed on the lining of the spinal cord.
- You may have developed arachnoiditis (see page 64).
- You might have lateral canal stenosis (see page 59).
- The area that was operated on may have become unstable, causing facet joint pain.

- If the operation was for a prolapsed disc, a second disc prolapse may have developed.
- In a fusion operation, the bones may not have fused solidly, a false joint may have developed between two segments of bone graft, or there could be a prolapsed disc above the fused level.

These problems occur in only five to ten per cent of patients who have surgery, but for some conditions the success rate is lower. About 20 per cent of fusion operations for spondylolisthesis result in the formation of a false joint. If spinal surgery fails to relieve your symptoms, the advice in the section on coping with pain (see pages 179 to 185) may be useful to you.

To reiterate, do not expect total and permanent relief from pain after an operation, or you are likely to be disappointed. If the operation is successful, and most are, the pain should certainly be dramatically reduced, and you should have much better mobility. To reap the greatest benefit, however, you must follow any advice given by the surgeon or the physiotherapist on how to look after your back, and you should use the self-help measures described in Chapters 13 and 14.

11
Acupuncture

For thousands of years, practitioners in the Far East have treated a wide variety of disorders by stimulating carefully selected points in the body with needles. Acupuncture was derided by most conventional Western doctors when they were first introduced to the practice about 200 years ago, and while many are still sceptical, orthodox medical circles are now beginning to recognize the value of this treatment. Since the early 1970s, there has been a huge upsurge of interest in acupuncture. However, the whole subject is rife with contradictory statements based on vested interests, wishful thinking and inadequate knowledge. It is difficult for a non-expert to cut through this jungle of research and opinions, and to find out whether acupuncture could be of any help in dealing with back pain. However, it becomes a little easier if you understand the traditional philosophy on which this form of medicine is based.

HEALTH AS HARMONY

According to the Chinese, good health was to be regarded as a state of energy balance within the body. They believed that the energy of life, which they called *chi*, consisted of a harmonious balance between the opposites *yin* and *yang*. Yin was seen as negative, cold, dark, passive, hidden, female and solid, while yang was positive, warm, light, active, open, male and hollow. Both were simply opposite ends of a continuous spectrum, and there is no definite cut off point between them.

The aim of Chinese medicine was to correct any imbalance in these forces, since this was the cause of disharmony or disease, and to allow the body's healing mechanisms to do the rest. The disease is, in effect, merely a symptom of an underlying energy imbalance.

The points and meridians
The ancient Chinese observed that certain areas of the skin became more sensitive when a particular organ or function of the body was impaired. These sensitive areas are known as points. The relationships between various internal organs and their functions were eventually synthesized into a comprehensive system of meridians. These are pathways which link all the points influencing a particular organ, and along which the energy of life flows.

There are 12 main meridians and two running down the front and back. Points along each meridian affect not only the major organ associated with it, but also other parts of the body which relate to that organ. Disorders of the nose and throat can be treated through points on the lung meridian, since they are involved in breathing. Points along the kidney meridian can influence organs that developed with the kidneys in the embryo: the testicles or ovaries and uterus. Each ear has an entire network of meridians and points, governing all the organs and functions of the body. The main meridians are reflected in three pairs of pulses at each wrist.

The aim of acupuncture is to identify the imbalance of energy which is causing the disease and, by inserting very fine needles at sensitive points along a particular meridian or meridians, to stimulate or reduce the energy flow until the harmonious balance is restored.

Ancient skill

Acupuncture is mentioned in the earliest recorded medical treatise, the *Nei Ching* or *Classic of Internal Medicine*, ascribed to the Yellow Emperor, Huang Ti, and supposedly written between 2697 and 2596 BC. There are also Chinese bone etchings which record the use of acupuncture in 1600 BC, while the Egyptian Papyrus Ebers of about 1550 BC refer to energy channels known to ancient Egyptian medicine and corresponding much more closely to the meridians of Chinese acupuncture than to the arteries, veins or nervous pathways of Western medicine.

The fact that acupuncture has survived through so many millennia suggests that it must have some genuinely beneficial effects; the problem comes in evaluating it. Because its roots are in ancient Chinese philosophy, orthodox Western medical criteria are, inevitably, clumsy tools for assessing its value.

THE MERIDIANS

Each meridian relates to a major organ and its functions; they are of different lengths, and each has a different number of influential points along it. For example, the heart meridian runs from the armpit to the finger tip and has nine points, while the bladder meridian runs from the forehead, round the back of the skull, down the back, and along the leg to the foot, and has 67 influential points along it.

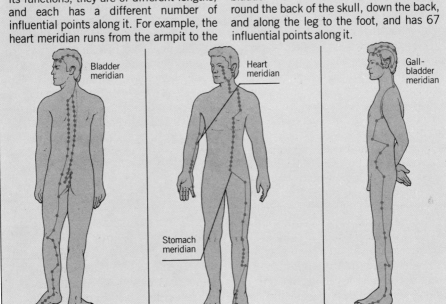

Bladder meridian

Heart meridian

Gall-bladder meridian

Stomach meridian

WILL ACUPUNCTURE HELP?

In general, acupuncture helps most back conditions by relieving pain and thereby reducing muscle tension and improving mobility. It does this through several mechanisms, including:

● local effects around the treatment point itself

● reflex nervous pathways between skin and muscle

● the release of pain-relieving hormones in the brain and spine

● blocking the transmission of pain either as it enters the spine or by preventing it from being relayed upwards to the brain.

Professor Ronald Melzack, an eminent researcher on pain, suggests that some chronic back pain may linger on long after the original reason for the pain, the damage to the back, has ceased to exist. Though your back may have recovered, "pain memories" have developed in the brain stem, rather like short circuits in an electrical system. He suggests that one effect of acupuncture could be to disrupt these short circuits and effectively switch them off, so that pain relief still persists long after the acupuncture stimulus has ceased. See Chapter 15 for a more detailed account of the psychology of pain.

Responsive personalities

Unfortunately, however, you cannot be guaranteed relief even if you have a condition of the spine which is potentially amenable to acupuncture. Many practitioners find that good results depend as much on the personality of the patient as on the medical condition: there are good responders and poor responders, and there is some interesting research to be carried out concerning which kinds of personality respond best to acupuncture.

A good responder does not have to believe in the treatment. He or she usually is decisive, impulsive, artistically or creatively inclined, and ready to take risks. A poor responder is the opposite.

Acupuncture and back pain

Supposing that you have the type of back pain, such as lumbago or sciatica, that might benefit from acupuncture, how can you tell whether or not it will really help in your case? One study in America shows that a great deal depends on the exact nature of your pain. Some 38 people who suffered from chronic lower back pain were tested with spinal injections of increasing strengths. Those whose pain could be blocked by relatively weak injections benefited from acupuncture: after seven half-hour treatments their pain was reduced on average by 63 per cent and the relief lasted for nearly four months. Those who needed stronger solutions of anaesthetic to stop the pain and those whose pain was identified as being psychological did not benefit to such an extent from their acupuncture treatments. People whose pain originated in the central brain structures, and those whose pain-conducting nerves had already been damaged, for example, in the course of operations, did not respond well to acupuncture. All this shows that there may be sound medical reasons why you may respond better or worse to acupuncture than your neighbour who has the same back problem.

The effective points

Other research is taking place to find out more about which acupuncture points work best. Some studies have compared the effects of treating acupuncture points and treating randomly

WHICH CONDITIONS RESPOND BEST?

We are beginning to understand more about how best to use acupuncture and what kind of back pain it helps most. In the meantime, if you have any of the problems which are listed here as benefiting from acupuncture, and if other treatments have not stopped your pain, acupuncture is very well worth trying. So long as the treatment is given by a well-qualified practitioner, acupuncture will certainly not be harmful. In so far as it is possible, I will attempt to list the conditions that may benefit.

Most likely to respond	■ Acute lumbago and acute wry neck — whether caused by a disc protrusion or facet joint problem ■ Wear and tear (osteoarthritis) of the facet joints ■ Episodes of acute pain due to instability in the lower back ■ Sciatica caused by disc prolapse (here acupuncture may be useful when other therapies, such as manipulation or injections, have failed) ■ Trigger point pain
Reasonably likely	■ Sciatica accompanied by signs of damage to the nerve root, such as weakness or numbess ■ Sacroiliac strain ■ Ankylosing spondylitis
Rather less likely	■ Agonizing sciatica with definite signs of nerve root damage ■ Severe brachialgia
Not to be considered	■ Central disc prolapse with sciatica in both legs, or bladder or bowel disturbance

selected points. The results show that both humans and animals can benefit just as much from treatment at non-acupuncture points as from treatment at traditional acupuncture points. Other studies show that simply needling trigger points, which are hypersensitive areas usually found within taut bands of muscle, can produce very good results, and it may be worth trying this if you suffer from trigger points (see page 49).

As research on back pain and acupuncture continues, the jigsaw puzzle of knowledge gradually produces a clearer picture of how much it can help back sufferers. Professor Chang Hsiag-Tung, of the world's leading acupuncture research centre, the Institute of Physiology in Shanghai, has said: "Traditional Chinese acupuncture, like many other things, is not all perfect, consisting naturally of both pearls and rubbish."

CONSULTING AN ACUPUNCTURIST

You may benefit from consulting an acupuncturist at any stage in your back condition, though it is wise to have a medical diagnosis first. Most people will have tried or been offered the more orthodox therapies before going to an acupuncturist and will consider an alternative in the following instances:

● When rest, analgesics, physiotherapy or manipulation are not helping to resolve an acute episode.

● To reduce pain and inflammation

arising from osteoarthritis in the facet joints which do not respond to improved posture, exercises or traction, or as an alternative to local injections to the joints or ligament sclerosant therapy (see pages 103 to 104).

● If you are suffering from chronic back pain or sciatica which is not amenable to surgery, or which has failed to be relieved by surgery, or for which you have declined surgery in favour of an alternative. In this instance acupuncture may help in certain conditions: for example, when painful trigger points have formed in the muscles adjacent to the affected spinal segments. When chronic "pain patterns" have set in, acupuncture may help to break the vicious cycle, perhaps by helping to close the pain gate (see page 176), relaxing the nervous system by controlling central pain pathways and by releasing the body's own pain-relieving hormones, the endorphins and encephalins (see page 177).

A few acupuncturists will refuse to treat conditions which they consider will not respond to acupuncture, but the majority will try to treat all patients who approach them.

Choosing an acupuncturist

In the United States and Britain there are recognized training colleges for the non-medical practitioner. Courses last three to four years and include academic study and clinical practice. It is advisable to select a practitioner who has a diploma from a reputable college (see Useful Addresses, page 187). The more experienced practitioner is probably also preferable to the beginner, as in any branch of medicine. Needless to say, you must choose someone you like and can communicate with, since very little in medicine that passes between the patient and the practitioner is purely a technical exercise.

More and more doctors are now practising acupuncture after learning the techniques on short courses. Although this arouses criticism and resentment among fully trained acupuncturists, research comparing the Western approach used by most of these doctors with the traditional Eastern approach has so far revealed no difference in terms of the effectiveness of the treatment.

My advice is to choose an acupuncturist who does have a more thorough background training and experience, but who is also medically qualified. These practitioners are obviously fewer in number, but they can draw upon all the resources available from both traditional acupuncture knowledge and modern medical expertise.

The diagnosis procedure

A traditional acupuncturist starts by trying to identify the imbalance which is causing the disorder, rather than diagnosing the exact nature of the illness: the disorder will disappear when the balance is restored. The diagnostic methods include observing the patient and asking questions, feeling various abdominal points and taking the pulses at the wrist.

Ideally, the skilful acupuncturist should be able to reach a diagnosis simply by feeling the pulses and without any other information. The pulses are also purported to register past and even potential future illnesses.

In practice, however, there are probably very few acupuncturists today in either the East or West who would rely solely on this method, if other methods of investigation are available. The President of the British Medical Acupuncture Society, Dr Felix Mann, advises that as a double check, one should "take a history, make a physical examination, laboratory investigations and so on, as

SELECTION OF POINTS

This depends on the probable causes of back pain which include:
■ Damage to soft tissue – disc, muscle and ligament injury
■ Degenerative changes in the bones and joints of the spine
■ Inflammatory conditions.

The points which may be used by the acupuncturist fall into several categories:
■ Local or adjacent points – traditional acupuncture points around the area that is most painful

■ Distal points – at a distance from the painful area
■ Influential points – points which govern a whole organ system
■ Tender points – not necessarily traditional acupuncture points, but points that are highly sensitive to pressure
■ Tonification – for the stimulation of energy
■ If the acupuncturist practises auricular acupuncture, he will select the relevant points on one or other ear.

suggested by the individual case."

In addition, the traditional style of careful examination and diagnosis along holistic lines is time-consuming, which poses problems for a busy acupuncturist, especially if he can obtain equally good results with treatment chosen on the basis of the patient's symptoms, his case history and a thorough knowledge of local acupuncture points.

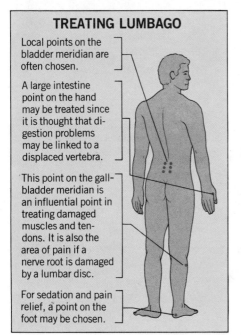

TREATING LUMBAGO

Local points on the bladder meridian are often chosen.

A large intestine point on the hand may be treated since it is thought that digestion problems may be linked to a displaced vertebra.

This point on the gall-bladder meridian is an influential point in treating damaged muscles and tendons. It is also the area of pain if a nerve root is damaged by a lumbar disc.

For sedation and pain relief, a point on the foot may be chosen.

The Western approach

As I talk to more and more acupuncturists of many different training backgrounds, it becomes clear that they all treat a patient with back pain in a very similar way, and that in the majority of cases the same treatment points will be selected, by whatever means the diagnosis was reached.

There are probably several reasons for this. In the first place, the chief symptom of most back trouble is pain. Whether the acupuncture points to deal with this are chosen because they relate generally to back problems or as the result of a detailed examination of the pulses, a sufficient proportion of patients find relief.

Secondly, musculo-skeletal problems are traditionally seen as falling into a somewhat different category from other illnesses, and are held to result not so much from energy imbalances as from disrupted meridians, so acupuncture points along these meridians are routinely chosen for needling.

On the other hand, an acupuncturist who is able to identify an underlying energy imbalance may choose distant points or meridians not generally associated with back pain. This might help patients whose back pain is not relieved after treatment at the normal points.

Some acupuncturists treat only through points in the ear, since there is an entire system on each ear which represents all the organs and functions of the body. This branch of acupuncture is known as auricular acupuncture.

Treatment

Once your acupuncturist has identified the relevant points, he will select the appropriate needles. There are various types of needle available in gold, silver or stainless steel according to the practitioner's preference. Most acupuncturists now use only stainless steel. The needles are extremely fine, much thinner than the usual medical hypodermic needle. The length of the needle varies with the depth of penetration required. The insertion of the needles may be entirely painless or it may produce a fine, stinging sensation that lasts no more than a second or two.

Once the needles are in place the acupuncturist will leave you to relax for ten to 15 minutes, which is the average duration of the treatment. You do not have to remain absolutely stationary but you will be encouraged to relax as much as possible. Sometimes, to adjust the

---

THE CONSULTATION

When you first consult an acupuncturist, he will take a detailed case history of your symptoms. He will also ask you questions about such things as your reaction to changes in the weather, and your food and drink preferences. Your answers provide information about your yin and yang make up, so that the acupuncturist can decide on the appropriate treatment to restore your yin and yang balance.

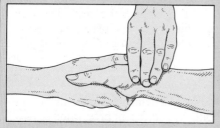

Taking your pulse (above)
The qualities of the 12 pulses at the wrist reveal a great deal about your health. The acupuncturist will spend several minutes feeling the pulses corresponding to the 12 main meridians. Apart from the health and speed of each pulse, he will feel for qualities such as whether they are hard or soft, rough or smooth, hollow or solid, and so on.

Receiving treatment (right)
You will need to lie down on a couch, and the acupuncturist will insert sterilized needles; the size of the needles and the depth of penetration will vary according to the energy imbalance. The finest needles are inserted with the help of a guide tube, because they are so fine that they would bend otherwise.

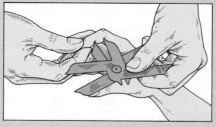

Locating the points (above)
When the acupuncturist has completed his diagnosis and decided which points to treat, he will locate the points either by touch or by using an instrument to calculate the "Chinese inch", a measurement unique to each patient.

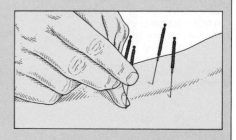

energy flow, he will twiddle the needles or gently pump them up and down.

The acupuncturist will probably use several needles. Once inserted they will produce a sensation known as *Teh Chi*, which is described as soreness, numbness, tingling or distension. It is not comfortable, but not painful either. If your problem is going to be helped by acupuncture, usually the degree and duration of improvement increases after each session. Eventually after perhaps a dozen or so sessions, the improvement reaches its maximum. Occasionally the symptoms are made temporarily worse by acupuncture treatment. Their aggravation usually resolves within hours or, at most, within a few days. If this happens, it often indicates that your problem will eventually be helped by acupuncture. If you have had no sign of improvement after two or three initial acupuncture sessions, the chances are that your condition will not respond.

ALTERNATIVE METHODS

Acupuncture points can be stimulated without using needles. Heat, pressure or a low electrical current can be used to adjust the energy flow instead of, or as well as, a needle.

Moxibustion

Chinese or Japanese trained acupuncturists may use a smouldering moxa stick, cone of moxa, or ball of moxa placed on the end of a needle, or directly on your skin. The moxa is removed when the sensation of heat is uncomfortable: it rarely burns the skin unless a small blister is the required effect. When it is placed on the end of a needle, heat is conducted down the shaft and produces a pleasant sensation which relieves pain and relaxes taut muscles. It clears the blocked channels and re-establishes the flow of chi energy.

Shiatsu or acupressure

Instead of using needles, some acupuncturists treat back pain by massaging the selected acupuncture points, particularly the tender points. Others will use some massage either before or after needling. The technique of massage is different from the Western method, which is primarily designed to relax the

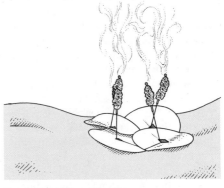

Treatment with moxibustion
Needles may be inserted into the relevant points and small cones of wormwood placed over them and ignited, card discs around the base will catch the ash (*above*). Alternatively, the acupuncturist will hold a lighted moxa roll over the point (*below*).

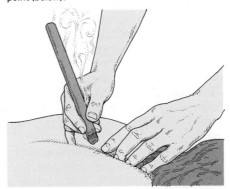

muscles and stimulate blood circulation (see page 172). Chinese and Japanese massage techniques are used in acupuncture to stimulate points or entire meridians with finger pressure, elbow pressure, stamping, scratching and so on. This massage may also involve mobilization of the spinal column on a par with osteopathy (see Chapter 8) or the Maitlands method (see page 83).

New equipment in acupuncture

All this equipment is intended for use by skilled therapists rather than home use. There are machines on the market called electro-acupuncture kits, which are claimed to detect the acupuncture points by finding areas that will conduct a current more easily. These areas are stimulated electrically using a probe that does not penetrate the skin. It has been shown, however, that if you rub a metal probe over the skin anywhere you eventually "sensitize" a small area, allowing the current to pass.

Even more recent is the introduction of laser acupuncture, a yet more impressive piece of apparatus which is claimed to fire a fine laser beam through a hand unit. A pulsing orange-red glow seems to pass through the target area of skin and the treatment is completed in a few seconds – without pricking the skin.

I have also seen an electrical recording device to measure the levels of yin and yang, simply by placing the measuring probe over a point on the meridian being investigated. The machine is supposed to monitor daily or even hourly fluctuations in these levels and record the response to treatment. If this was genuinely validated, however, I should think that all acupuncturists seriously concerned with evaluating their treatment would be using one by now.

Although I may sound somewhat sceptical about the benefits of this new

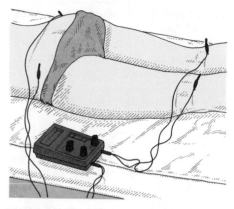

Electronic acupuncture
Acupuncture points can be stimulated by a low-voltage electrical current. Acupuncture needles are inserted and electrodes are then attached to the ends. The current is switched on and gradually increased until the patient is just able to feel it. The points used above are for treating sciatica.

acupuncture compared with the traditional methods of needling, the face of modern acupuncture is changing very fast. On some courses, practitioners are now trained in the use of equipment that measures "energy imbalance" in the upper and lower halves of the body. This is designed to help them plan their treatment more appropriately.

A further new development is the use of an electrical current for stimulation through the tip of a needle. Electrodes are attached to the needle and the patient holds another electrode in one hand to complete the circuit. This is thought to be more efficacious in some instances than traditional methods of twiddling the needle.

In summary, it seems that there are many ways of stimulating these points and whichever method is used there is potential benefit. Unfortunately, there is not enough evidence available at present to state clearly which method of stimulating the points is more effective than the others.

12
Alternative therapies

If you have tried one or more of the treatments already discussed and found them wanting, or if they do not offer much hope in your particular case, perhaps one of the therapies covered in this chapter will prove useful.

They are all based on holistic principles, treating you as a person rather than just isolating your back as a specific problem. Most of the therapies discussed in this chapter emphasize the interaction between the mind and the body. Some, such as the Alexander technique and homeopathy, treat the body directly with physical remedies. Others, including hypnotherapy, meditation and bioenergetics, tackle physical symptoms by altering mental attitudes.

Whichever method you decide to try, it is important to choose an instructor or therapist with whom you can establish a good rapport. If you like and trust your therapist, and have faith in his ability to help you, the treatment is more likely to succeed. Your attitude towards any therapy you receive is very important, and can affect its outcome.

Emotional problems as a cause of back pain have already been mentioned (see page 14), and the relationship between mental attitudes and pain perception will be discussed in Chapter 15 (see pages 175 to 178). There can be no doubt that the mind has considerable power over the body, and can influence it for good or ill.

HYPNOTHERAPY

Although this does not offer a cure for your condition, hypnotherapy will be able to help you by influencing your perception of pain. Under hypnosis, your control over your conscious mind is suspended temporarily, so that your subconscious thoughts, feelings and memories can be reached. The hypnotist can help you gain access to completely subconscious functions in your brain, such as the translation of messages from your nervous system into feelings of pain. In this way, the hypnotist can give you the power to control your perception of pain. Even when you come out of the hypnotic trance and are fully conscious again, the pain will be considerably reduced.

Not all people respond equally well to hypnosis. The most suitable patients are people who are able to let go, to trust others and, of course, to relax. It is essential that you are willing to accept the ideas presented by the hypnotist. It would be impossible for you to be persuaded to do something against your will, even if you were in a deep trance. If you are unable to respond effectively to hypnotherapy, you may still be able to benefit from a form of self-hypnosis (see opposite).

As with most therapies, you have to strike a balance between expecting nothing, and expecting too much – which inevitably leads to disappointment. If you have chronic back pain, it is not going to vanish merely because the hypnotist suggests this. It may decrease, but the main aim for someone in chronic pain is to help him relax, and to improve his confidence and ability to cope.

Procedure

In the first session, the therapist will take a full history of your symptoms, and ask various questions to discover

HYPNOTHERAPY AND CHRONIC BACK PAIN

A study undertaken in San Francisco in 1977 gives a clear illustration of the way in which hypnotherapy can help someone with chronic back pain. Eight people, who had all been in pain for between one and 23 years, were given between eight and 14 hourly sessions of hypnosis.

Initially, they were all given relaxation training in order to reduce their muscular tension, and increase their body awareness. This was followed up and reinforced by further instructions in self-awareness, combined with breathing exercises.

During the subsequent individual sessions of hypnosis, the therapist guided each patient back in imagined time, temporarily erasing his personal memories, and also forwards, temporarily removing personal expectations of the future. The training then moved on to thoughts and images associated with calmness, relaxation and peace.

Once the patient was thoroughly relaxed, the hypnosis was deepened. The hypnotist encouraged the patient to discover which particular thoughts, feelings or images were reliably associated with deep relaxation. After this, he would be asked to visualize the colour, size, shape, temperature and location which he associated with the various aspects of the pain.

The idea of this was to show the patients how to reduce the pain by producing thoughts, images or feelings which were incompatible with it. For example, a patient might imagine an ice-pack being placed over or around the burning sensation which was part of the pain. Using this technique, the patients were trained to raise or lower the pain level, proving the extent of their own control. Once one painful sensation, such as burning, had been eliminated, they could move on to the next aspect, for example, throbbing, stabbing or twisting, and tackle that in the same manner.

The final element of training was to teach each person how to extend what he had learned, so that he could use his newly acquired skills to control the level of his pain in a wide variety of situations when he was fully conscious.

Four months after this treatment the eight patients were still in much less pain. They were able to sleep better and to enjoy a more active social life. They were less dissatisfied with their lives and less depressed. However, there was no improvement in their ability to engage in sports or in sexual activity. Nevertheless, they exhibited fewer of the personality characteristics associated with chronic pain, such as hypochondriasis and hysteria (see page 178), and they took fewer pain-killers. Bearing in mind that all of these people had been in chronic pain for between one and 23 years, and no other medical treatments had been successful, the results suggest that hypnotherapy is well worth considering as a treatment for anyone suffering from chronic pain.

whether you are anxious or depressed and to assess your motivation towards recovery. He will give you a full account of what is involved in later sessions.

In the next session, the therapist will sit close to you, usually facing you, and will talk you into the trance state, perhaps asking you to focus your eyes on a particular object. When the therapist feels that you are sufficiently deeply hypnotized, he may simply tell you directly that your symptoms will clear up. Alternatively, he might question you, to explore possible reasons for your health problems.

In later sessions it is often much easier and quicker to become hypnotized, and the effect may be achieved merely by the hypnotist counting down from ten or snapping his fingers.

SELF-HYPNOSIS

A milder state of hypnosis can be self-imposed. The technique is a type of auto-suggestion, but it should be learned from a professional hypnotherapist.

You will learn to relax thoroughly, perhaps using a method similar to that given on page 171, or by repeating instructions to relax different parts of your body, for example "My arms are heavy; my legs are limp." You will be encouraged to focus your attention on certain bodily sensations, particularly your breathing rhythm.

When you are thoroughly relaxed, physically and mentally, your mind will be receptive to new concepts. You will be taught to introduce ideas which create a new image of yourself as being fit, healthy and free of pain. With practice, you will be able to retain this new self-image for long periods. Even when you come out of this state of utter relaxation, you will benefit from mental tranquillity and greater self-confidence, which are important factors in helping to reduce your back pain.

MEDITATION

Although meditation may not sound like a therapy for back pain, it is closely allied to self-hypnosis, relaxation training (see page 171) and, in some ways, to psychotherapy. As there is a psychological element to all pain (see Chapter 15), regular meditation can help you to recognize and reduce stress in your body, and to overcome the anxieties and fears that are causing the stress.

The aim of meditation is to bring the mind under control and focus it in such a way that you are freed from all stressful fears and emotions. Dr Herbert Benson of the Harvard Medical School has discovered that meditation also lowers the heart beat and respiration rates. In addition to this, it tends to synchronize and harmonize the electrical patterns produced by the brain, inducing alpha brain-waves, which generally indicate a calm mind.

Most people will benefit from regular meditation. It is particularly useful for back sufferers whose muscles are chronically tense, and who are very anxious. Both of these states may be major factors in causing the pain. Additionally, people in chronic pain may find that meditation helps them to cope with it.

Types of meditation

There are many different forms of meditation and it is much easier to learn initially from a teacher. In many areas there are local centres or groups who will teach you the basic techniques, and there are even some family physicians who run meditation groups in their own practices and health centres. If no teacher is accessible, you can try the method described below, which combines several meditation practices.

If you decide to go to a teacher, how do you know which type of meditation is most suitable for you? This depends partly on your personality and the state of your back, and partly on your own personal choice. The active forms of meditation, of which Rajneesh is the best known, involve spontaneous movement, adopting various postures, deep breathing and facial contortions. If you have an acutely painful back, this may not be the best choice for you. On the other hand, if you have recurrent back pain which is partly the result of postural tension, this method may help you to loosen up, emotionally and physically. The more passive forms of meditation

include transcendental, Buddhist and yoga techniques. In the first, you will be led into a higher or transcendental state of consciousness through the silent rhythmic repetition of a word or sound. In yoga or Buddhist meditation, you will concentrate on a single object or thought, focusing your mind and attempting to watch thoughts and reactions without emotion. The attempt to do this is often aided by complex breathing techniques, and the aim is to reach a state in which perception of yourself and all personal desires are lost in a sense of unity with the universe.

If all this seems a far cry from back pain, just remember that a lot of people develop back trouble precisely because they are too bogged down and involved with their own activities and emotions: most people benefit from mental tranquillity, especially back sufferers.

SIMPLE MEDITATION METHOD

■ Choose a quiet room with no distracting noises such as television, radio or music.

■ Sit or lie down, in whichever position you find most comfortable and effortless.

■ Start by closing your eyes and relaxing all your muscles (see page 171), but do not worry about how deeply you are relaxed; this will come with time and practice and if you start worrying about it you will probably tense up anyway.

■ Breathe through your nose. Become aware of your breathing, and as you breathe out say the word "one", silently and slowly, to yourself. Breathe easily and naturally for ten to 20 minutes. Do not dwell on distracting thoughts, attempt to ignore them and return to repeating "one".

■ When you finish, sit or lie quietly for several more minutes, first with your eyes closed and then with them open.

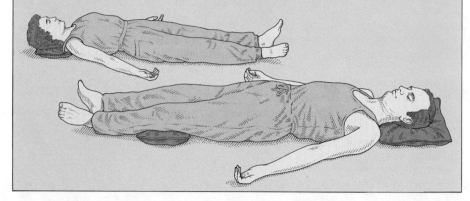

THE ALEXANDER TECHNIQUE

This aims to treat and prevent a whole range of disorders by improving posture. The Alexander technique is based on the principle of relaxing muscles – particularly the neck and shoulder muscles – and of adopting the posture that puts least stress on your spine.

An Australian actor, F. Matthias Alexander, developed this technique towards the end of the nineteenth century, after retiring temporarily from his acting career due to the sudden and inexplicable loss of his voice during performances. Doctors were unable to help him, so he diagnosed his own problem. He discovered that, just before delivering any speech on stage, he pulled his head backwards and downwards in a manner which cut off his voice. From this discovery, he went on to form the Alexander principle.

He differs from the founders of osteopathy and chiropractic in that he did not regard vertebral malalignment or a reduction in mobility as problems to be tackled by themselves. He maintained that they were due primarily to misuse, and believed that habit and use dictate function. Our posture exerts a constant influence on general function, physiologically and psychologically. The influence of the body on the mind and of the mind on the body cannot be separated.

The Alexander technique is not a method that you can learn on your own; you must go to a qualified teacher. We all have a unique posture, just as our fingerprints and voiceprints are also unique. Because of this, the Alexander technique can be taught only on a one to one basis, and the set of lessons may be very different according to what is required. All pupils are taught techniques developed specifically for their own posture, which should be practised every day. The course may involve just five or six lessons over a few weeks, or it can last up to a year.

Procedure

The Alexander teacher may work with you sitting, standing or lying, depending on what he feels is required. Your teacher may start by watching you as you change position from sitting to standing. You will be encouraged to imagine that you are being pulled upwards from the crown of your head. A key theme is to visualize the kind of posture that you would have if you were in full health and strength, and to maintain the image in order to achieve this type of posture.

People who have learned the Alexander method commonly say that it is a question of undoing all the habits that have become second nature. In the lessons they often feel that they are being asked to adopt postures and positions which feel entirely unnatural because over the years their bad posture has grown to feel more natural to them than good posture.

SUCCESS STORIES

John Dewey, the American educationalist, studied the Alexander method because he had been clumsy all his life. He credited the technique with benefiting his health, as well as improving his posture and generally increasing his awareness of his own bodily activities.

Aldous Huxley, who was another student of the Alexander method, described it as a comprehensive system of physical education that achieves a heightening of consciousness at all levels, and is a way "to prevent the body from slipping back under the influence of greedy end-gaining into its old habits of mal-coordination."

THE ALEXANDER TECHNIQUE

The Alexander teacher will help you to eliminate postural defects by studying the way you sit, stand and move. The lessons will be tailored to your unique posture.

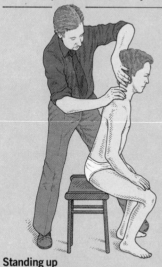

Standing up
The teacher will show you how to keep your spine straight when you stand up rather than leaning forwards and pulling your head back.

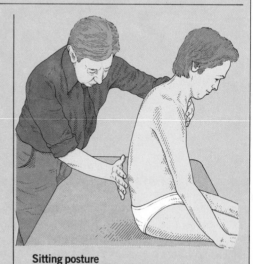

Sitting posture
The teacher will help you to achieve good sitting posture by encouraging the right amount of curve in your lower and mid back and neck.

Suitable cases

Almost everyone has some postural defect, and could benefit from a course of the Alexander principle. Most people who attend these courses, however, either suffer from some intermittent or recurrent backache or neckache, or feel generally under-par. The course will not cure acute problems such as a disc prolapse or malaligned facet joints; however, once an acute attack is over, the Alexander technique will certainly help to prevent a recurrence. It is especially useful for avoiding postural pain, and in elderly people it may prevent acute episodes of back pain by teaching them to use their backs carefully.

FELDENKRAIS TECHNIQUE

This therapy is similar to the Alexander technique, and, like the Alexander method, it claims to promote general health by improving posture. Moshe Feldenkrais, a Russian-born Israeli who trained as a physicist and engineer in Paris, believed that altering someone's postural habits would affect his personality. "The bulk of stimuli arriving at the nervous system is from muscular activity constantly affected by gravity," he wrote, "so posture is one of the best clues not only to evolution but also to the activity of the brain."

The technique can be taught to groups of people or to individuals on a one to one basis. The most suitable cases are people with postural defects and those with chronic back or neck pain caused by tension. Dancers, actors and athletes, who need flexibility combined with physical fitness, may also benefit from this therapy.

BIOENERGETICS

Another therapy that is based on the principle that our posture reflects our mental state is bioenergetics. Unlike the methods developed by Alexander and Feldenkrais, which try to alter mental attitudes by improving posture, this therapy tackles the mind directly through a form of psychotherapy developed by Dr Wilhelm Reich, a pupil of Sigmund Freud.

Personality types

Reich believed that children develop through three overlapping phases, for example the "oral phase" between birth and 18 months of age is overlapped by the "anal phase" which lasts until the child is about 24 months old. During the third stage, the "genital phase", the child begins to develop independence and contact with external reality. Biologically, it is the anchoring of the energy focus in the genitals, and children start to show a stronger interest in those parts between two and four years of age.

If psychological development is arrested during any of these stages, certain characteristics remain dominant in the personality. Intellectual and physical development may continue quite normally, but the person's emotional outlook on life is immature.

The "oral character", for example, remains dependent on other people and in particular on his mother. He is dissatisfied, believes that the world owes him a living, and feels too weak to achieve things for himself. His slack posture and weak muscles cause backache and shallow breathing, and his rounded shoulders lead to neck pain.

The "masochistic character" has arrested psychological development during the "anal phase". He identifies with the underdog, and feels both his own

and other people's suffering intensely. The upper half of his trunk tends to sag downwards, and the muscles in his neck and pelvis are tight, particularly around the throat and the rectum. Typically the person's face has a mask-like expression and his voice is whining. He tends to be overweight, with a heavy pelvis.

Other personality types include rigid characters, whose behavioural patterns developed as a result of frustration or suppression during the "genital phase". Examples are the "hysterical" female who over-reacts emotionally and dramatizes situations, and the compulsive military commander type, obsessed with punctuality, tidiness, perfection and over-control of his environment. Most people are a mixture of many types, but often one type predominates.

The language of the body

The posture associated with any of these personalities may result in backache due, for example, to chronically tense muscles. Any restrained impulses lead to physical and mental stress, and suppressing the reaction to a single childhood trauma can cause chronic tension. The typical "masochistic character" described above is constantly suppressing anger, which keeps his or her muscles contracted and tense. Other personalities have characteristic patterns of tension in the body which frequently lead to back pain, or, like the "oral personality", are characterized by slack posture. By resolving inner conflicts and releasing suppressed emotions, bioenergetics reduces this tension, and can thus eliminate back pain.

The therapy

Based on the principle that personality is determined by development during childhood, the therapist makes use of a variety of methods to understand a patient's behaviour. The therapist will encourage you to talk freely about your childhood, your parents, your dreams and fantasies, in order to gain access to your deeper feelings. Your therapist may ask you to adopt a position which imposes some stress in your body, or to perform deep breathing exercises, in the hope that this will mobilize suppressed emotions such as anger, sorrow or joy. If, for example, he finds that the oral character is dominant in your personality, he will help you to construct a more positive self-image and to mobilize your aggressive impulse by becoming more self-assertive. If he discovers that suppressed emotions are contributing to your pain, he will encourage you to express those emotions, physically or vocally. This will help you to dispel the tension in your body.

Deciding to consult a therapist

Anyone with back pain caused by postural defects might benefit from this therapy, particularly those in chronic pain who are prone to anxiety or depression. It is available only from a private psychotherapist who has been trained in these methods and who has undergone this therapeutic process himself. The therapy is usually given in a series of one hour sessions every week or two over a few months.

HOMEOPATHY

Homeopathic medicine is based on the principle that "like cures like". In the eighteenth century, a German doctor, Hahnemann, noticed that certain natural drugs derived from plants and chemicals reproduced exactly the symptoms of certain diseases if they were given to healthy people. He discovered that these same drugs cured the diseases whose symptoms they reproduced.

Further investigation of the phenomenon revealed that more dilute mixtures are much more potent treatments than concentrated mixtures. For this reason, the drugs are always given in extremely dilute doses – perhaps one part active ingredient to 200,000 parts diluting substance. Homeopaths argue that their treatment is much safer and freer from side effects than conventional medicine, due to the dilution of their drugs. The remedies can be given as tablets, liquids, powders or ointments.

The mechanism involved in homeopathy cannot yet be explained – the remedies probably work by stimulating the body's natural defence system – however, it is well established that the treatment does work, and can be used preventatively too. It has been used successfully to help rheumatoid arthritis patients in the homeopathic hospitals in Glasgow, Scotland.

Homeopathy and back pain

Homeopathic remedies can be used to treat a number of back conditions, including sciatica, lumbago, stiff neck and strained ligaments or muscles. A large number of chemists stock homeopathic remedies, and since the drugs are very safe due to the dilute doses, many can be bought without a prescription.

Consulting a homeopath

A major difference between conventional treatment and homeopathy is that there is a wide variety of homeopathic drugs to treat a single condition, each suited to a particular type of person. If you consult a homeopath, he will ask not only about your symptoms, but also about apparently unconnected factors such as what type of weather you like, and if you prefer to stay up late or get up early. Even the colour of your hair and your personality are factors in determining which drugs are suitable for you. In this way, the practitioner will form a picture of your physiological and psychological constitution, and will choose a drug to suit you.

Homeopaths are trained for four years before they are qualified to practise. Some family practitioners are trained in homeopathy as well as conventional medicine, and will offer homeopathic treatment to their patients.

FOOD ALLERGY

Most of the types of back pain described so far in this book are caused by well-defined conditions. However, a small number of people suffer from widespread and varying symptoms related to the back, which are not easily diagnosed. Research by two doctors in the United States suggests that symptoms such as headaches, tense muscles, joint pains and general fatigue can be caused by an allergy to certain foods. Such allergies usually produce intermittent symptoms relating to several different systems in the body. A typical example would include widespread muscular and joint pains, stiffness, headaches, dizzy spells, impaired balance, irritability and fluctuating moods. Recent studies in the US suggest that rheumatoid arthritis may be affected partly by diet.

The exact nature of the mechanisms that produce these reactions is not fully understood, but it is well established that these chronic conditions can sometimes be completely cured by excluding certain common foods, such as milk products or wheat products, from the diet. A few people have mild allergies to a range of fruits, vegetables, meats, colourings, preservatives or beverages. Some people are even allergic to certain chemicals in ordinary tap water, or to some minerals which are dissolved into food from cooking utensils.

Allergy testing
The most effective way of testing for a food allergy is to fast for five days on spring water only, and then introduce particular foods one by one. This must be done under medical supervision, because a five-day fast can be very taxing, and any allergic reactions developing after the fast can be much more severe than the previous symptoms.

Usually, if your condition is related to your diet, all your symptoms will have cleared up by the third or fourth day of your fast. After the fifth day, you will be advised by the specialist to introduce certain foods and drinks which are the most common causes of allergic symptoms – such as milk, wheat products, sugar, coffee, or an individual fruit or vegetable. If one of these produces your symptoms again, you should eliminate it from your diet.

CASE HISTORY
A railway worker in his early forties came to me with a history of pains around the neck, shoulder blade and chest area. His case had been dismissed as psychosomatic after investigations showed nothing wrong, but he realized that he might have a food allergy. He tested various foods, and as soon as he cut out all dairy products from his diet, his symptoms vanished.

13

Posture and everyday activities

A great deal of chronic or recurring back pain is due to poor posture, and in a way this is heartening, because everyone can do something about their posture without recourse to drugs, surgery or other drastic measures. The way in which we stand, sit and move is to some extent laid down genetically in terms of the structure of the skeleton and the flexibility of the joints. In addition, children copy their parents: there is often a striking similarity in the gait and posture of parents and their children.

The remainder of postural development, however, is a combination of various factors which affect us from birth onwards, including illnesses and injuries, fitness, nutrition, physical activities and, last but by no means least, our personality and outlook on life.

Changing your posture
Assuming that your back trouble is at least in part caused by your posture, what can you do to alter the latter? You may be able to change your posture for a minute or two if you concentrate, but this temporary change is unlikely to banish backache. Posture that has developed over many years tends to remain fixed, but with perseverance you can alter these fixed muscular patterns.

Poor posture often reflects underlying depression and low self-esteem. Sometimes, the state of mind that is reflected in poor posture is stronger than the desire to transform that posture, but at least it is well worth making the effort to change, because success will bring mental as well as physical rewards.

There are two ways in which you can approach the problem: either you start by changing your mental attitude, perhaps with the help of meditation techniques (see page 130), in the hope that your posture will improve with it; or you try to alter your posture and maybe this will produce a marked change in your mental attitude. The real challenge is carrying this improvement over into your everyday life, when you cannot always be thinking about your physical posture and mental attitude.

Matthias Alexander developed a comprehensive programme which teaches good posture and educates us how to move without straining our backs. The Alexander technique is described fully on page 131.

Be aware of your posture
If you are going to try to change your postural habits, you need to think about the muscles you use – for the most part

subconsciously – to support your spine, and the different ways in which they are brought into play. In order to avoid back trouble, you need to be aware of the best posture both when you are moving and when you are still. It is all too easy to strain your back simply by standing wrongly, sitting on a badly designed chair, leaning over a desk, or sleeping on a mattress that should have been thrown out years ago.

Static postural stress

Your spine is under considerable stress if you stay in a bad position for a long time. Static posture typically results in tense, aching muscles, and painful ligaments. To avoid this type of back pain, it is essential to adopt a posture which minimizes stress on your back and lets your muscles relax, whether you are standing, sitting or lying down. You should also move around occasionally.

STANDING POSTURE

There is no single ideal posture, since people come in all shapes and sizes. The ideal posture for you is one in which your back is put under the least strain, and in which the spine is curved naturally and gracefully. The essence of good posture is fitness – if you keep your muscles well toned and supple, you stand a good chance of achieving the correct posture for you, especially if you can reinforce this with a relaxed mental and emotional state.

How to avoid bad posture

In the context of back pain, bad posture means any posture that puts your spine

RECOGNIZING POOR POSTURE

In good posture, muscles are relaxed without being slack, and the spine itself is gently S-shaped. In poor posture, the muscles are either too slack or excessively rigid, and the spine has exaggerated curves or is held too stiff and straight.

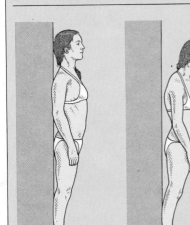

Rigid posture (far left)
The traditional military-style posture, with the back stiff and straight and the chest out, is fatiguing and restricts normal breathing. It produces a lot of muscle tension around the neck, shoulder, mid and lower back areas and restricts the upper abdominal muscles and diaphragm.

Slack posture or sway back (left)
The head and chin hang low and the neck pokes forwards. Upper back and shoulders are rounded. The muscles supporting the spinal column and abdomen are slack. If the rigid posture looks uptight and aggressive, this looks hangdog and submissive. Sway backed posture is common among overweight people. If you have a beer paunch or are in the latter stages of pregnancy, you will be carrying a lot of weight in front of you. This puts extra strain on the back, leading to an exaggerated curve in the lower back and a forward-tilted pelvis.

STANDING PELVIC TILT

If your bad postural habits are deeply ingrained, this exercise may not be easy to begin with, but persevere with it. Try the pelvic tilt lying down at first (see page 157) if you cannot manage it standing up. Good posture will gradually become more natural, until holding your pelvis correctly is no longer an exercise, but a way of life.

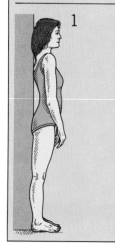
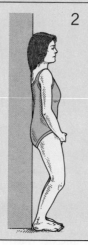

1 Stand with your back to a wall, so that the hollow is clearly defined.

2 Keeping your shoulders against the wall, bend your knees slightly and flatten your lower back against the wall by tightening your abdominal muscles and drawing your pubic bone forwards.

3 Practise the movement regularly and concentrate on getting the correct angle. When you can do this easily, you need not stand against a wall to do it, and can try it with your legs straight.

under unnecessary strain. Although by "poor posture" we generally mean slack posture, an excessively rigid posture can be equally bad for the back. This results in tense muscles and may even restrict your breathing. It is not surprising that soldiers faint sometimes if standing to attention for any length of time. If you suffer from aching shoulders and neck, try to relax these muscles, and do not adopt a rigid stance.

If you are carrying a lot of weight in front, the stress on your spine is increased, not only because your pelvis is tilted forwards unnaturally but also because your centre of gravity is moved further forwards. As a consequence, the back muscles have to work harder, which increases the compression in the lower back.

It is important to strengthen your abdominal muscles and – if possible – to lose weight. If you are overweight and cannot easily go on a diet, you may find that a corset will help to reduce back pain by providing extra support for your spine. This should be only a temporary measure, as a corset is no substitute for firm abdominal muscles.

If you are pregnant, try to hold yourself as well as possible and make sure that your work surfaces are the right height (see page 147), so that you do not have to stoop. Avoid wearing high heels, which can lead to a hollow back even when you are not pregnant.

Standing correctly

A major feature of overweight or slack posture is that the pelvis is tilted forwards, which produces a hollow back. You should try to set the pelvis at the correct angle so that the lower back has a normal, slight curve, rather than an unnatural hollowed-out appearance which puts the lower back under stress.

When you are busy it is easy to forget to tuck your pelvis in all the time. When standing, try resting one foot on a low stool or foot-rail about 10 to 15cm (4 to 6in) above the floor. This relaxes the psoas muscle, which stretches from the lower back over the pelvis to the thigh, thus altering the angle between the lower back and the pelvis. You will find that it relieves stress with no undue muscular effort, and the technique can easily be used at work and in the home.

SITTING POSTURE

All of us put our backs at increased risk of stress if we spend long hours sitting every day. Just a glance at the figures below based on a chart produced by an eminent researcher on back pain, Alf Nachemson, will tell the story.

Sitting imposes more strain on the spine than standing or walking, and as soon as we begin to lean forwards more than a few degrees the pressure increases dramatically. If you have to sit down for a long time, a comfortable, well-designed chair can reduce the risk of back or neck pain and headache.

The ideal sitting position

For anyone who spends a lot of time sitting down, a well designed chair is an essential part of back care. Your chair should be fully adjustable so that you can alter it to suit your measurements.

Although the "perfect chair" includes a slight curve for the lower back, there is considerable debate among the experts over how much support is needed for the lower back. Some hold that it must have substantial support, while others believe that a straighter or even a slightly concave shape is preferable. The best shape for you may depend on the cause of your back pain, and what you will be doing when using the chair. You should try out several types before deciding which is the best for you.

Sitting at a desk

If you are working at a keyboard or typewriter, your chair seat is probably best kept horizontal and you will need firm support for your lower back. To avoid stress in your neck and shoulders, the desk or table should be at a height which allows your fingers to touch the keys with your arms bent just slightly

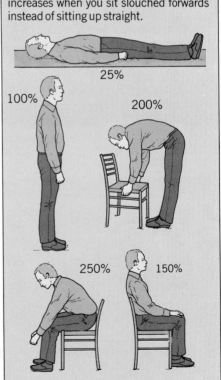

PRESSURE ON THE SPINE
Pressure within the lumbar discs is defined as being 100 per cent when you stand up straight. Note how much it increases when you sit slouched forwards instead of sitting up straight.

25%

100%

200%

250%   150%

below the horizontal, or your chair should be adjusted to that height. However, if you get low back pain, it is more important to keep your chair at the correct height for the length of your legs. You should be close enough to the machine to work without stretching your arms forwards from the shoulders.

If you have to spend long periods leaning over a desk, it is best to have a sloping work surface so that you do not need to bend your head and neck down. You may also prefer a seat that can be tilted forwards slightly. This decreases pressure on the spine, and means that you need not bend your neck so far.

Even if you spend much of your working day typing or leaning over a desk, you should change position regularly, and take breaks from time to time to avoid backache. An ergonomically designed office chair (one adapted to the needs of your body) should have a seat that is adjustable in height and can tilt downwards to allow you to lean forwards, for example, to reach for the telephone. It should also be able to tilt

backwards so that you can relax into a semi-reclining position, during a pause for thought, perhaps. The backrest should be adjustable, and the best ones tilt forwards or backwards according to the angle of the seat.

Head and neck alignment

If your back is rounded or you are frequently involved in work that entails leaning over a work surface with your head bent forwards, the muscles in your upper back, shoulders and neck can easily become fatigued. The result can be a painful neck or headaches – migraine can be induced by chronic neck tension. Whenever your neck feels tense or you find that you are holding your head forwards with your chin out, try to reduce the curve in your neck by pulling your chin back and making the crown of your head the highest point.

The neck retraction exercise described on page 164 reduces tension by bringing the weight of your head more directly over your spine, so that your neck muscles have less work to do.

CHOOSING A SUITABLE CHAIR

The dimensions of your chair should suit your body measurements. The ideal dimensions are given below: if your chair does not correspond to these, you should adjust it, or use cushions to bring it up to the correct height or to support your back.

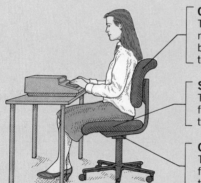

Chair back
The back of the chair is upright, but very slightly moulded to support the natural arch of the lower back, and it is high and broad enough to support the full width of the shoulders.

Seat depth
The depth of the seat is sufficient to support the full length of the thighs – if it were any deeper the back would be left unsupported.

Chair height
The seat is at a height which allows the feet to be firmly placed on the floor with the thighs horizontal and the lower legs perpendicular.

THE BALANS CHAIR

Originally designed in Denmark, the Balans chair is now becoming very popular for use in the home and in the office. It helps to make you aware of the position of your spine from moment to moment. Although it is almost as easy to slouch and round your lower back in this chair as in any other, you will probably be more aware that you are doing it. Obviously this type of chair is not comfortable for people with knee problems, and even if your knees are healthy this chair takes some getting used to. Those who have persevered tend to be very enthusiastic.

Advantages of the Balans chair
The spine is held erect with just the right amount of curve. Body weight is transferred away from the pelvic bones, down the thighs and on to the knees. This dissipates some of the compression at the base of the spine which can contribute to lower backache.

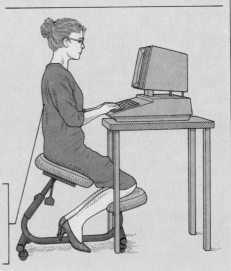

Relaxing in a chair

Good sitting posture does not mean sitting up straight for long periods. You must relax in order to avoid straining muscles. If you watch anyone attempting to sit bolt upright, you will notice that after about ten minutes he or she will slip into a relaxed, slouched position. When you are relaxing at home, you need a comfortable chair with enough space to allow you to change posture: if you are to avoid strained, tense muscles you must be able to move around while you watch television or read. Cushions behind your lower back will help to support your spine.

Rocking chairs prevent you from sitting still for too long. The gentle exercise is soothing and helps to relieve backache, for example, in pregnancy and you can use it later to rock your child to sleep.

DRIVING

If you have a bad back, driving can be agonizing unless you have a good car seat and well placed controls. Important factors to consider are: clear vision (obviously, safety has to come first); that the controls are within easy reach; that your arms and legs are relaxed and that your body is properly supported.

When you are driving, get into the habit of relaxing your neck and shoulder muscles. Try to become aware of times when you grip the wheel too tightly or hold it too high up and with your arms outstretched. Notice whether your shoulders are hunching up towards your ears: if they are, develop a relaxed and steady breathing rhythm, and with each breath let go of your tight muscles, slowly dropping your shoulders. Gently work your head and neck back into a more relaxed position, and make use of your headrest.

The car seat

The cushioning of a car seat is very important, too. It must not slope towards the middle, or too much weight will be borne by the pelvic bones instead of the thighs. In addition, it must be firm enough to resist the indirect forces when you use the pedals. If the seat is too hard, as used to be the case with tractors, vibration from the engine is transmitted up to the spine, which can cause back problems.

The foot pedals

Foot pedals should not be too high off the floor, and should be directly in front of the seat rather than to one side. The clutch should not be too stiff. Car manufacturers frequently appear to make the chauvinistic assumption that all large cars will be driven by men. If you are a small or average height woman, the foot controls may be too far apart or incorrectly angled for your feet; the strain of operating them, particularly in heavy town traffic, can lead to back pain. If you have experienced this with your car, it would be worth investigating the possiblity of having the pedals changed.

The backrest

The backrest of a driver's seat should give good support to the lower back, both lengthways and sideways. Some car seats now have an adjustable lumbar bar which you can position to suit your back. Alternatively, you can buy cushions for the lower back which can be attached to the backrest by a strap. It is important that you can alter the angle of the backrest: the optimum angle is between five and ten degrees behind the vertical. You should also be able to adjust the height of the seat, though not so much that it affects your vision and control of the car.

The headrest

You should be able to rest your head comfortably on the headrest, relaxing your neck and shoulder muscles, while still looking straight ahead. The headrest should be slightly padded, and adjustable both up and down, and forwards and backwards.

Special problems

For some people, such as airline pilots, whose jobs entail sitting for prolonged periods, moulded backrests can prevent back pain. Tailor-made to each individual's spine, these backrests are made of fibre-glass resin covered in a cushioned material and are very lightweight and portable. The British Air Force has successfully reduced back pain in aircrew by providing them with this type of individually made support.

LYING DOWN

Many back sufferers find that they are most comfortable lying down, though once again there are no hard-and-fast rules. If you feel your typical back pain developing and you know that it will be relieved if you lie flat for five or ten minutes, then by all means do this. When you lie down, you are relieving your spine of a great deal of the weight of your body and this will reduce the compression on, for example, a protruding disc. It is not, however, essential that you lie flat: experiment with some of the positions shown in Chapter 5 (see page 69) until you find the one which is most restful for you.

If your back pain is at its worst in the morning, you might be wondering

whether you should change your bed.
If this is the only time your back aches,
there may indeed be some connection,
but often aching and stiffness is just the
result of several hours of inactivity, and
it may not make much difference which
surface you lie on. It may not be just a
coincidence, though, if this waking pain
has developed only since you bought a
new mattress.

So-called orthopaedic beds, which
are custom built, cannot be truly tailored to the individual on the basis of the
few details that are taken. Any finely
sprung mattress which supports you
should be adequate, and may save you
some money. You should sleep on a bed
that is at least 15cm (6in) longer than
you, to allow freedom of movement.
Ultimately, however, your bed is very
much a matter of individual taste: some
people prefer very hard surfaces, while
others can get a really good night's sleep
only on a soft bed. Stick to what you
find most comfortable – you are the one
who knows best whether or not it is
harming your back.

The mattress
If your mattress is too soft, it will not
support your body sufficiently, so that
when you sleep your ligaments and joints
will be under strain and will become
painful. A good mattress should be firm
and should contour itself to your body.
It does not need to be excessively hard,
but it should not sag.

The bed base
A bed base that has lost its spring or is
sagging can harm your back. If your
bed base is sagging, try putting a board
under the mattress to make it a little
firmer. It need not run from head to foot
but it must cover the whole width of the
bed at least as far down as the level
where your buttocks will lie.

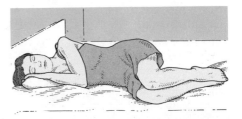

Foetal position
You may be more comfortable if you lie on your
side in the foetal position with your knees and hips
bent at a comfortable angle.

POSITIONS TO LIE IN
Lying on your front increases the curve
in the lower back and this will aggravate
backache due to facet joint problems.
This position will probably not hurt
your back if your pain is caused by a
prolapsed disc. See page 69 for more
detailed advice on comfortable positions
during an acute attack.

For most people, lying flat on their
backs with their legs straight out also
tends to increase the curve in the lower
back and cause backache. The Fowler
position, with your legs supported so
that your knees are bent, helps to flatten
out the excessive curve and also relaxes
the psoas muscles, which run from the
lower back to the thighs. If you have
acute back pain, you may need several
pillows under your knees (see page 69),
but otherwise a rolled-up towel may be
all you require.

Avoiding neck pain
To avoid neck pain, you need to make
sure that your head can rest fairly square
on your shoulders, whether you lie on
your back or your side, so that the strain
will be minimized. To achieve this, you
will probably need one pillow if you are
lying on your back. If you sleep on your
side, the width of your shoulders will
determine whether you require one or
two pillows to support your head.

PILLOWS

An old, floppy pillow is not going to give your head sufficient support. To test whether a pillow is in good order, lift it up horizontally, with the edge of your hand running across the centre. If the pillow stays more or less level, all is well. If it sags down over your hand, buy a new one.

If you frequently wake up with a stiff neck, try twisting a pillow into a butterfly shape or even use a rolled and twisted towel to act as a soft collar (see page 69). This gives your neck the extra support it may need, and prevents your head lolling from side to side as you sleep. You could also try one of the various special pillows designed for back/neck sufferers, such as the one illustrated on the right.

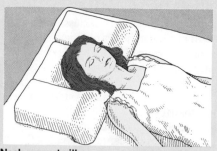

Neck support pillow

This pillow is rolled under at the front to hold the neck and head firmly and put a very mild traction on the neck. It is divided into three sections, the two sides are slightly higher to support your head properly when you are lying on your side.

ADAPTING YOUR ENVIRONMENT

If you suffer from backache, it makes sense to analyze your activities at work and at home. When considering your job or tasks to be done at home, ask yourself the following questions:
● Can the effort be minimized – for example, by asking for help?
● Will you need to stand in an awkward position for any length of time?
● Does the task entail repetitive movements such as bending and twisting? If so, you will be taking a considerable risk and should work only for short periods at a time, with intervals of rest in between.
● Is the task very strenuous? If so, you may become very tired and more prone to strain or injury.
● Do you know how to lift and carry things properly?
● Is there any constant postural stress involved as, for instance, in hanging wallpaper, cleaning windows or painting a ceiling?
● Is there repetitive stress, for example,

the bumping entailed in driving heavy vehicles over rough ground?

From the answers to these questions you can decide whether it would be more sensible to stay away from work or put the job off until you feel better. If you decide that the job is feasible, plan it out following the guidelines given below. Above all, concentrate on the job. If your mind is on other things, or if you are performing your task under pressure, you are likely to be distracted from the immediate job. This increases the risk of back injury. Anger or frustration with the task itself is also rather distracting, and the added tension will make you more liable to back injury.
● Try to anticipate any pitfalls before beginning the job: for example, is the ground uneven? Are you likely to slip or fall? If so, clear the ground first or work out a safer route.
● Wear appropriate clothing: if you are wearing smart clothes you might hold objects away from your body, which

LIFTING TECHNIQUES

When you lift anything, even if it is light, you should avoid bending your back. Always take the weight on your strong leg muscles rather than your back muscles.

LIFTING A BOX

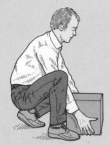

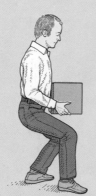

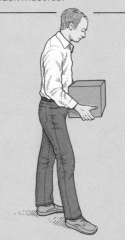

1 Squat down on your haunches with one foot slightly in front of the other and the object between your knees. Grasp the object firmly: place one hand underneath it with that arm straight, and use the other arm to steady it. Grip with your whole hands, not just your fingers.

2 Keep your back straight and lean forwards very slightly. Stand up in a single, smooth movement, keeping the object close to your body and taking the weight on your legs, not on your back. Make sure that you do not bend your back as you stand up.

3 When you carry the object, always keep its weight close to you. Put it down in reverse order: with one leg slightly in front of the other, squat down without bending your back.

LIFTING A LONG LOAD

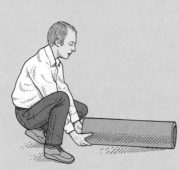

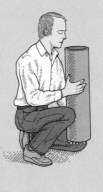

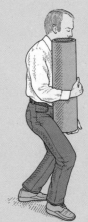

1 Squat down with one leg in front of the other and one end of the load between your feet. Put both hands under the end nearest you.

2 Raise just one end of the load, until it is vertical, and rest it against your shoulder. Shift one hand if necessary to prevent the load toppling over.

3 Grip the load firmly underneath with your other hand. Stand up, keeping your back straight, and taking the weight on your legs.

protects your clothes but puts extra stress on your back.

● Make sure that you are able to stand properly with adequate space around you and without stooping.

● Make sure that you grip an object firmly before lifting it; use a sling or ropes if necessary.

● Keep a straight back whenever you lift anything.

● Keep the load close to your body and tuck in your pelvis to minimize stress on the spine.

● Lean with your back against heavy objects to move them, instead of pushing with your arms.

● Buy any tools that will help you to do the task more easily.

● Avoid unnecessary effort: put objects on a suitable work surface so that you do not have to stoop; use a trolley or other transport device to save you some effort. If you can lift the object easily with one hand, use the other to provide support and stability.

● Divide the load into smaller loads. If you can't, don't try to move it.

● Use other parts of the body instead of your back to take the weight such as the shoulders, pelvis or thighs.

● If the object does not have to be put down gently, drop it.

Lifting and handling techniques are especially important for the worker in heavy industry. Training has dramatically reduced the incidence of back injury in some settings. However, we all do a lot of lifting and carrying every day, and whether you are doing the housework, shopping, or gardening, you are likely to spend a substantial proportion of your day lifting and carrying, and a little forethought and planning may save you a lot of pain.

When you are going on holiday, for example, bear in mind that it is easier to carry things if you are balanced on both sides, so use two small suitcases rather than one large one, perhaps with a rucksack on your back. The alternative is to use strap-on casters, which need fairly large wheels for negotiating steps, plus a good handle on the suitcase. The same principle applies to shopping: divide your purchases evenly into two smaller loads or use a trolley. Putting heavy objects into the back of the car can be difficult and may strain your back, so try to get help, or restrict yourself to small, manageable loads.

PLANNING THE HOME

Much of the work involved in running a house is stressful for back sufferers, but the problems can be minimized with careful planning. Wherever possible, adapt your environment to reduce stress and strain on your back.

The kitchen

Since a great deal of housework is centred on the kitchen, an ergonomically designed room will pay dividends. Kitchen work tops all tend to be the same height, so adjustments may have to be made. For most jobs, the work top should be slightly lower than your elbow, with the exception of the sink, which needs to be at elbow height. If you share the work with someone else, you might consider having a work top each. If necessary, the units can be raised on a plinth.

If your sink is so low that you have to stoop to wash up, use a bowl and raise it to the right level by putting it on a stand or an upturned bowl. When standing at a sink or work top, rest one foot on a low stool or foot-rail.

Store heavy objects, such as casserole dishes, at working height and within easy reach, so that you do not have to bend awkwardly or stretch to pull them out whenever you need them.

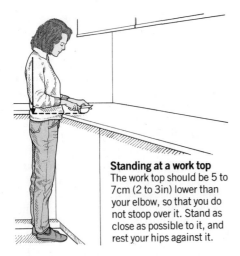

Standing at a work top
The work top should be 5 to 7cm (2 to 3in) lower than your elbow, so that you do not stoop over it. Stand as close as possible to it, and rest your hips against it.

The bathroom

Like the kitchen, the bathroom is a place where a little planning can save a lot of backache. After you get up in the morning your back is quite vulnerable. Simply standing and leaning forwards to shave with your arms held high may initiate stress in the back, heralding the start of a bad day. To avoid this, put the mirror to one side of the basin so that you can stand close to it, or use an extendible mirror.

When washing your hair, do not bend over the basin but kneel down by the bath and use a shower hose. When bathing, especially when you have an acutely painful back, take care not to lie with your back in a rounded position for too long. You may be comfortable in the bath but you could be in trouble when you get out. A hand rail half-way along the side of the bath is useful if you have chronic back trouble.

HOUSEWORK

Everyday chores around the house can be very hard on the back. If you have chronic back pain and can't get help with the housework, work out a rota so that you do not have lots of strenuous tasks on any one day. Do not try to clean the house in one go: there is no point in being a martyr. Do one room and then have a rest. In general, avoid prolonged and repetitive tasks. Try to alternate these jobs so that at least there is variation in the types of stress and strain on your back.

Washing clothes

Hand-washing clothes can be very hard work. As with dish washing, make sure that your sink is not too low; if it is, use a bowl, either on a stand in the sink or on the draining board. If you are using a sink or basin, pull out the plug and let the water drain away, then press some of the water out of the clothes before trying to lift them: this will save wear and tear on your clothes as well as on your back, because wet cloth is very heavy and can tear from its own weight.

When you are emptying your washing machine, put your basket on a low chair or stool and transfer the clothes at that level. You will not have so far to lift them later on. When hanging up your washing, make sure that the line is at a sensible height, so that you are not continually straining upwards. Keep the basket on a chair and your clothes pegs handy. Use a line prop or pulley to raise and lower the line.

Ironing

This can be a strain, particularly if you cannot adjust your board to a comfortable height. It should be low enough for you to lock your elbow (in other words your elbow should not be bent up at an angle of less than 90 degrees), but high enough so that you do not have to stoop. Unfortunately, the standard maximum height for ironing boards is 90cm (36in), so if you are tall you might be better off with an ironing board hinged to the wall at an appropriate height.

Bed making

This is inevitably a strain for back sufferers. If you have a family, train them to make their own beds, or if this is not possible, find ways around the problem. For example, buy fitted sheets and duvets, which are less trouble than flat sheets and blankets. Squat down or kneel by the bed instead of bending over when you tuck in the sheets. The higher the bed, the better, as you will not need to bend over so much. Unfortunately, the current trend is for lower and lower beds. Make sure that the bed is on smooth-running casters so that you can move it around easily.

Cleaning

Use brushes and brooms with long handles to minimize bending. Lean against them to use the weight of your body rather than just your arm muscles. To vacuum under low objects, kneel on one knee and keep your spine straight instead of bending from the waist. Bending over to clean the bath can cause back injury, so use a long handled brush and kneel beside the bath. Encourage your family to clean the bath after they have used it. Kneel down to wash the floor. For windows, use long-handled tools so that you do not have to stretch.

GARDENING

Many tasks in the garden involve crouching or bending for a prolonged period, both of which can aggravate back problems. Other jobs entail lifting heavy loads, which can be equally dangerous, especially if this is the only manual work or exercise you undertake and your muscles are out of condition.

In general, the basic advice on back care, and in particular on lifting and carrying, applies. Work in an upright position as much as possible, using your body weight rather than your muscles whenever you can, for example when digging. Do not do too much at once, and change tasks often, to reduce the number of repetitive stresses that can fatigue muscles and ligaments.

Garden tools

You can help yourself a great deal by ensuring that you have good tools. For example, if you have a motor mower which needs to be started by a cord pull, make sure that the cord is long enough and the mechanism is not too stiff. When using a mower, push the machine rather than pull it, since this will impose less strain on your back.

Wheelbarrows are a mixed blessing: they are often badly designed, so that the weight of the load does not lie over the wheel as it should, and there is a natural tendency to overload them. Lifting a heavy, ill-balanced load onto a wheelbarrow and then pushing the barrow over soft ground, twisting to stop the load tipping to one side when you hit an unexpected bump: what could be a better recipe for a prolapsed disc? If you must use a wheelbarrow, make sure that it is not too large or heavy and is built to carry the weight over the wheel rather than near the handles. Avoid overloading it and use it only for essential tasks: grass cuttings, for example, are better placed on a polythene sheet and pulled to the compost heap.

Make sure that hoes, rakes and other implements have long enough handles; try to use them in the most energy-saving way and establish a comfortable rhythm; do not carry on for too long.

For crouching and bending activities, use long-handled trowels and forks, avoid pulling actions, and use rubber knee pads or mats. If you cannot kneel, it may be necessary to convert your garden to raised borders or to grow plants on shelves in the greenhouse.

WORKING IN THE GARDEN

These activities can be agonizing unless you take care. There are now several digging tools on the market which have been designed for people with bad backs, including the semi-automatic spade. The golden rule when digging, however, is to choose the right time. If the earth is wet and heavy, you will put quite unnecessary strain on your back. If the ground is hard, dry and compacted, the same applies. Finally, if you have a bad back and you know the soil is full of stubborn roots and has not been tackled for years, persuade someone else to do it for you, even if you have to pay them.

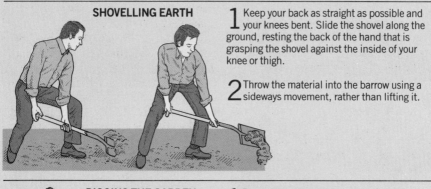

SHOVELLING EARTH

1 Keep your back as straight as possible and your knees bent. Slide the shovel along the ground, resting the back of the hand that is grasping the shovel against the inside of your knee or thigh.

2 Throw the material into the barrow using a sideways movement, rather than lifting it.

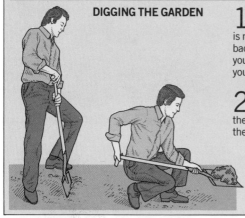

DIGGING THE GARDEN

1 Do not grip the spade any tighter than necessary, and work at a steady, even pace: there is no point in rushing the job and wrecking your back. Keep your back straight and bend from your knees. Push the spade into the ground using your body weight, not your muscle power.

2 Cut around the sides of each spadeful before you start to lift the soil. Hold the handle at the end and use the spade as a lever to ease out the soil.

3 Raise the soil by holding the shaft of the spade near its base. Do not lift too much at one go, and turn it over as soon as you can, rather than wasting effort and straining your back by lifting it too high.

CARING FOR CHILDREN OR INVALIDS

Looking after young children or caring for the elderly involves a lot of lifting, carrying and stooping over beds. Pay special attention to your lifting technique, and watch out for snags: children may struggle, and elderly people may be unexpectedly heavy. Many people with small children are particularly prone to back trouble.

BABIES AND TODDLERS

Children are not the sole cause of back trouble, but they certainly constitute a risk. This is especially true for women.

During pregnancy, natural hormonal changes lead to a softening and stretching of the ligaments of the spine and pelvis. It takes up to five months for these ligaments to tighten up again after the birth, so if you are a new mother, you will be particularly vulnerable to developing back strain from weak and over-stretched stomach muscles, poor posture or faulty lifting.

For a man with a bad back, the problems are more likely to come from the fact that most baby items are adjusted to the height of an average-to-small woman. You may want to be fully involved in caring for your baby, but not if it means stooping over baby baths and nappy-changing tables designed for someone a head shorter than you. Fortunately, there are simple ways round all these problems.

Washing and changing a baby

You do not need to use a special nappy-changing unit; the important thing is to do the job on a work surface that is the right height (a little below elbow level, as for kitchen work tops) such as a chest of drawers. Alternatively, kneel on the floor and then change your baby on a low bed or settee. Similarly, you should bath your baby at a comfortable height – perhaps on one of the kitchen work surfaces. Fill the bath in pan loads, and empty it this way as well, until you can carrying it easily to the sink or basin.

Lifting and carrying a baby

Choose a cot with a side that can be lowered right down, since this saves you bending over to pick up the baby. Lower the side of the cot as far as it will go, squat down beside it and pick up the baby. Rise up from your haunches, keeping the baby's weight close to you. Take care when lifting your baby out of the cot: if he or she is struggling, or if a piece of clothing or a foot catches on something, there may be an unexpected tug on your back.

Carry your baby in a special baby carrier on your back to distribute his or her weight close to your centre of gravity. Baby slings worn at the front are useful, but they tend to slacken and impose a strain similar to that of pregnancy, except that the baby is now somewhat heavier.

If you suffer from back trouble, try to get help when lifting a carrycot or find ways around the problem. If possible, carry the cot and the baby in two separate trips. If you cannot find anyone to help you, stand on one side of the cot, bend your knees, keeping your spine

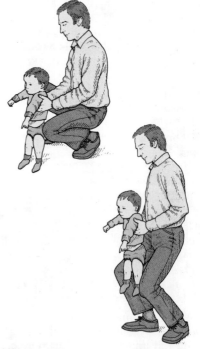

Lifting a child
When you lift a child, follow the basic rules of lifting: squat down by the child and use your leg muscles to rise up again, keeping your back straight as you stand up.

straight, and lift the cot carefully, keeping its weight close to your body. If you are pushing your baby in a pram or a push-chair, ensure that the handles are long enough, or buy extension handles.

If you have a bad back, it is obviously unwise to swing a child around at arm's length, however tempting this may be. Pause and think before you undertake any activity: a bad back may be a considerable source of discomfort and irritation, and if this is not appreciated you may find that you are unloading some resentment on your child without realizing it. Remember that your child will be happiest when you are happy. Careful forethought and a well-planned environment will make parenthood and babyhood much more enjoyable.

CARING FOR INVALIDS

If looking after a baby can strain your back, caring for an elderly parent or invalid is obviously going to put your back at risk. Avoid problems by making sure that all the surfaces which the invalid uses are on much the same level. This will enable you to slide him or her from the bed on to a chair and then on to a commode. You can obtain sliding platforms with handles, which make this much easier. Use a cantilevered bed table and raise the bed on blocks so that you do not have to bend over whenever you need to lift the patient. You can buy special hoists to lift or lower the patient, although you will probably need some training from the suppliers to learn how to use them properly.

SEXUAL ACTIVITY

Sexual function can certainly be limited in an acute attack of back pain, but the problem is much more serious for the chronic sufferer if pelvic movements are painful. Sometimes back pain may be used as an excuse to avoid sex, although this may be entirely subconscious and the sufferer will probably deny it.

Most couples with a loving and physically warm relationship will find ways around any restriction on their sexual life. In fact the pelvic thrusting movements in sex may work very well as a mobilizing exercise while you are recovering from an acute attack. Notice the similarity between love-making and the exercises shown on pages 157 and 159. If acute back pain develops while having sex, the most likely cause of the pain is dislodged or strained facet joints. It should be relieved by gentle pelvic tilting (see page 157) to flatten the curve in your lower back and reduce strain on your facet joints.

Comfortable positions

If you have facet joint strain, you will probably be better off on your back with your partner on top. If both partners are unfortunate enough to have back problems, lying side by side may be preferable. If your partner is much heavier than you and your favourite position is lying on your back, it may be worthwhile trying a change while your back is aching. For a woman with backache, the all-fours position with the man entering from the rear, may be more comfortable, but do not arch your back too much. A man with severe back pain may be more comfortable sitting on a chair with the woman astride him. In this position the man is relatively passive and the woman is able to move more freely.

The most important thing to emphasize is that there are very few illnesses which should be allowed to interfere totally with physical intimacy between two loving partners. There are some useful booklets on fulfilling sexual activity produced for the disabled and paraplegics. They all emphasize the importance of touch, communication, tenderness and emotional intimacy. It is often necessary to distract one's focus from the usual goals of genital satisfaction and orgasm, since these may prove too frustrating. Quite often this advice is given by sex therapists to physically normal and healthy couples who are having sexual difficulties. There is more than a grain of truth in the statement, generally accepted by sex therapists, that sexual pleasure is 90 per cent mental and only 10 per cent physical.

Pelvic block

There is a possible link between sex, posture and back pain which could prove an interesting area for research. I have noticed that some back sufferers have enormous difficulty learning to perform the pelvic tilt, which is the basis of a sexual movement. This observation raises the question: just how comfortable are they with their own sexual impulse? In psychotherapeutic circles this inability is given the name "pelvic block", and I suspect that, with some people, there is a link between their sexual identity and stiffness in the lumbar and pelvic region, which may predispose them to back pain.

SPORTS

Most sportsmen have their fair share of back injuries, but it is difficult to identify particular sports which carry a much greater risk of back problems. There are, however, certain movements or activities in sports which may aggravate existing problems. If you are prone to recurrent backache, be alert for any warning signs such as sharp twinges or an intermittent ache. When you notice these signs, avoid any sport such as golf, hockey, squash or football, which involves vigorous twisting, turning or bending, and redouble your preventative exercises (see pages 157 to 162).

Warming up

You must always do warming-up exercises before any sport: cycling for five to ten minutes on an exercise machine, jogging on the spot for a similar period or the "patter" routine. This is a form of jogging on the spot: keep your toes on the ground and lift your heels alternately, raising your knees only a few centimetres, as rapidly as possible.

Once your pulse rate has been raised a little (you will be able to feel your heart beating faster), you should perform stretching exercises appropriate to your sport for another five or ten minutes (see pages 160 to 162). It is important that the following muscles are stretched before you start your particular sport.

● For any sport that involves running – the calf muscles and Achilles tendons, see stretching exercise on page 161.

● All sports – hamstring and quadriceps muscles (the muscles at the back and front of the thighs), see stretching exercises on pages 161 and 162.

● All sports – back muscles, but exercise gently and take care not to overstrain them (see page 169).

● All running sports – groin and inner thigh area. Stand with your legs apart, point your right foot outwards, bend your knee, and squat down keeping your left leg straight and both feet flat on the ground. Hold this position for a few seconds, then repeat on the other side. Alternate ten times.

● Particularly racquet sports – trunk muscles by gentle twisting movements, see exercise on page 160.

● All sports – shoulder and shoulder girdle area, by swinging your arms.

After a period of vigorous exercise you should cool down, repeating the stretches which you did at the start. If you follow these guidelines, you will reduce the risk of strains while you are participating in the sport, and you will not feel so stiff afterwards. Your spine will also benefit from these routines.

High risk sports

For certain sports you will be able to reduce the risk of injuring your spine if you take care to ensure that particular muscle groups are kept in good trim. Golf, for example, involves a vigorous twisting and turning movement, which imposes considerable stress on the lower back. To counteract this, your spine needs good muscular support, particularly from the muscles which run down and across the abdomen (see page 12).

Serving in tennis or badminton and bowling in cricket entail a combination of overhead action and trunk twisting, which can put an excessive stress on the facet joints in the lower part of the spine. If you have been training too hard or your technique is poor, these joints can become inflamed and irritated, particularly if there is a difference of more than a centimetre in the length of your legs. The problem can often be solved if you modify a faulty technique, take a brief period of rest and practise some muscle strengthening exercises (see pages 166 to 170).

Long distance running can impose stress on the joints of the lower half of the body, including the spinal joints. People running considerable distances, say 80 to 100 km (50 to 60 miles) a week, may sustain stress fractures due to overuse. If these have been identified by X-ray, you will have to rest until they have healed. You may avoid this type of injury by ensuring that your hamstring and lower back muscles are stretched regularly, since they tend to tighten rather easily in runners. Check, too, on the angle at which you tilt your pelvis (see page 138). Wear well-padded running shoes, and avoid jogging on hard surfaces, such as roads or pavements, in order to minimize the jarring effect on your spine. Try to keep level ground, since running up or down hills adds to the stress on your spine.

Another cause of back trouble in runners is the habit of swinging the arms repetitively across the body. This rotates the trunk to and fro on the facet joints of the lower back, which are basically designed to restrict rotation. As you run, try not to swing your arms across your front too much.

Whatever the sport, it helps to be fit. Fatigued muscles play a part in a great many sports injuries to the back, since anyone who is not really fit and who tires early on in a game is risking some form of injury.

General fitness

Fitness is important not only to those who play sport, but also to relatively inactive people. If you are fit, a good, relaxed posture probably comes naturally. If you have recurring back pain caused by poor posture, it is well worth taking up exercises to make you fit, once an episode of acute pain has died down. You will then be able to reach up and stretch, or to carry things, without undue effort, so you will be less likely to injure yourself by straining or holding yourself awkwardly. If you do hurt yourself, the damage will probably be less severe, and your general fitness will help you recover more quickly.

14

Exercise and massage

Exercising your back is an important element in recovering from acute backache, and may well help those who have chronic back pain. Some of the exercises suggested here are designed to help with specific back problems, while others are for general back care. The strengthening exercises may prevent a recurrence of back trouble, or help you to avoid back pain altogether.

The step-by-step instructions for each exercise in this chapter should enable you to do the exercises on your own without any expert supervision. If you are not sure whether you are doing them correctly, ask a professional, such as your physician or physiotherapist, to watch you. Use the chart overleaf to help you decide which exercises are the most appropriate to your condition, and start with the more gentle exercises. Stop if any of them increases your pain.

One of the best forms of exercise for general fitness and mobility is swimming. The only stroke that may aggravate backache is the breast stroke, due to the tendency to arch the spine in order to keep the head above water. Otherwise, swimming is a beneficial aerobic activity which exercises most of the large muscle groups and stimulates the circulation. It also flexes the joints without any risk of straining them, because the water supports your weight and resists excessive movement.

Cycling is another way of maintaining general fitness while recovering from an episode of back pain. This will not jar the spine in the way that running can. It is preferable to use a bicycle that does not have drop handlebars, because the racing position is too flexed: the old-fashioned upright position puts less of a strain on your back.

Exercising after an acute attack
After an acute attack, you should begin exercises as soon as you can move without undue pain. However, it cannot be stressed too emphatically that if any exercise increases your back pain, you should stop doing it at once. On the other hand, when you start exercising muscles that you have previously neglected, you are likely to feel the normal aching and slight stiffness which this entails, and you should not let this mild discomfort put you off. If you are in any doubt as to whether the exercise is beneficial or not, seek expert advice.

Exercise prescription
I have not laid down rules about how frequently you should perform any of

the exercises given in this chapter. People vary greatly in the amount of time and effort which they wish to contribute. In general, while you are recovering from an acute attack, do a few of these exercises at least daily, and they should ideally be done two or three times a day. I have recommended the number of repetitions that the average person can manage. Do not worry if you can manage only two or three repetitions to start with. As you become fitter, repeat the exercise 20 or even 30 times

per session. Most of the specific therapeutic exercises give most benefit if performed as often as ten repetitions every couple of hours throughout the day.

You need no special equipment for any of these exercises, just a little space. Some of them can even be done at work. Wear loose, comfortable clothing, but you do not need special sports clothes. At work, just loosen your belt or your tie so that your movements are not restricted. Do not try any exercises immediately after a large meal.

RELIEVING BACK PAIN WITH GYNAECOLOGICAL CAUSES

Gentle exercise is very effective in relieving back pain during menstruation or pregnancy.

Menstruation

Young girls sometimes experience acute backache associated with the onset of menstruation. Usually, exercise such as walking, cycling or swimming relieves it, alternatively, an early night with a hot water bottle is a comforting relief. Aching joints may be caused by fluid retention, so eating a healthy diet and cutting down on fluid intake the week before your period is due may help. Deep relaxation (see page 171) will help to reduce your pain, especially if you practise it regularly the week before your period starts. There are a few gentle exercises that may also help. Practise them the week before your period is due, and for the first couple of days of menstruation.

■ Lie on your back on the floor with your knees bent up and your feet on the floor (see Pelvic tilt, page 157).

■ Kneel on all fours and hunch and sag your back alternately. See Mountain and sag exercise, page 159.

■ Lie on your stomach over a low stool and make swimming movements with your limbs, as if you were doing the breast stroke.

Pregnancy

Many women experience backache in pregnancy, most commonly in the last three months. This is often caused by poor posture (see page 137) and slack ligaments (see page 47). If you are pregnant, you should pay careful attention to your posture, particularly to the angle at which you hold your pelvis. The pelvic tilt (see page 157) done either standing up or lying down, will help you to avoid sway-backed posture, and the standing extension exercise (see page 159) may relieve your pain. Since your ligaments will be softening up throughout your pregnancy in preparation for the birth of your child, you must be careful of the way you lift and carry objects throughout pregnancy, and for the first few months after the birth, to avoid ligament strain and joint malalignment (see pages 44 to 47). Chapter 13 offers advice on correct lifting and handling technique and some tips on posture. You may find that some of the following positions help to relieve backache during pregnancy.

■ Sit cross-legged

■ Lie on your back on the floor with your legs straight up and slightly apart, supported against a wall

■ Sit on the floor with your legs straight out in front of you and slightly apart

■ Squat on your haunches

■ Stand about three feet away from a wall with your legs a shoulder width apart. Place your hands at waist height on the wall, with your back horizontal and your legs straight.

CHOOSING THE RIGHT EXERCISE

If you are suffering from an episode of acute back pain, start with the appropriate exercises in the left hand column as soon as you can move without too much pain — probably about a day after the attack began.

Progress to the exercises in the middle column when the severe pain has subsided. The exercises in the third column are stretching and strengthening exercises which may help you to avoid back trouble.

Condition	During acute attack	When severe pain has gone	Prevention
Acute and chronic lumbar pain (caused by disc or facet joint)	Pelvic tilt Passive extension* Mountain and sag	Passive extension* Standing extension Low back stretch* Side gliding Gentle twisting Side bending	Hamstring stretches Abdominal exercises Leg exercises
Acute wry neck (caused by disc or facet joint)	Passive extension	Neck retraction Passive extension	—
Acute pain in the leg	Pelvic tilt Passive extension*	Passive extension* Low back stretch* Gentle twisting	Hamstring stretches Abdominal exercises Leg exercises
Lumbar instability	Pelvic tilt	Passive extension Low back stretch	Abdominal exercises Leg exercises
Facet joint disease	Pelvic tilt	Low back stretch	Abdominal exercises
Strained muscles	—	Gentle twisting Side bending Low back stretch	—
Tense muscles	Low back stretch Gentle twisting Side bending Calf stretch Hamstring stretches Neck retraction Neck stretch	—	—
Trigger points	Specific exercises to stretch the affected muscles	—	—

*If your pain increases after six repetitions, do not continue the exercise

LOWER BACK EXERCISES

These exercises may help you if you have acute pain in the lower back, whatever its cause, or sciatica. If you have consulted a doctor or physiotherapist, you may have been given instructions about exercising your back, and you should follow this advice. But if you have recurrent attacks and are familiar with the exercises, or if you feel that your attack is not sufficiently severe to warrant a consultation, then it may be worth trying any of the following exercises. Begin the exercises about a day after the pain first started, but stop at once if the pain is increased or spreads away from your spine.

PELVIC TILT

This movement is of general benefit in most types of acute lumbar pain regardless of the specific cause. It relieves pressure on the facet joints and gently stretches the muscles and ligaments of the back. It may stimulate the local blood circulation, and it undoubtedly strengthens the abdominal muscles, which indirectly support the spine. If practised regularly, it encourages better posture, which will help to prevent back pain. Do this exercise lying on the floor to start with, but later on try the same movement standing up. If you find it easier, you can do the exercise with your legs supported on cushions in the Fowler position, see page 69.

PASSIVE EXTENSION

This exercise is beneficial to many kinds of backache which are brought on by sitting. Try it only if you can lie face down without increasing your pain. If bending backwards or regaining the upright position is difficult because you are already stuck in a stooped position, lower yourself slowly until you are lying face down, and relax in this position for a few minutes before starting the exercise. Try the exercise two or three times initially: if the pain increases during it or shortly afterwards, or if it seems to spread further away from the spine rather than towards it, this is not the exercise for you. If you have sciatic pain which is made worse by it, avoid this exercise.

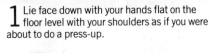

1 Lie face down with your hands flat on the floor level with your shoulders as if you were about to do a press-up.

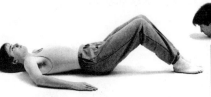

1 Lie on the floor with your arms at your sides, your feet flat on the floor and your legs bent at a comfortable angle.

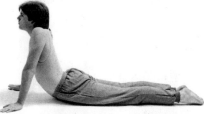

2 Push up with your arms, leaving your hips on the floor. Lift your head and shoulders as high as you can, and let your back sag in.

3 Breathe out, then slowly lower your trunk, using your arm muscles only. Repeat up to ten times, allowing your spine to arch progressively more with each repetition.

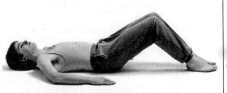

2 Gently press the back of your waist against the floor and tilt your pelvis forwards by tightening your abdominal and buttock muscles. Hold this position for at least six seconds, then relax slowly. Repeat up to ten times.

SIDE GLIDING

The side gliding exercise was developed by the physiotherapist Robin Mackenzie, to help people with acute lumbago who have a tilted pelvis or a list to one side, often due to a disc protrusion or an acute facet joint strain. If it causes increasing pain in the back or legs, stop immediately and ask the advice of your therapist.

Look in a mirror to see which of your hips is more prominent. If it is your right hip, your lower spine is leaning to the left, and this exercise should help you to pull your pelvis towards the left, and glide your trunk to the right, as shown below. If your left hip is more prominent, perform this exercise the opposite way round.

1 Stand with your feet a shoulder width apart, your knees straight and your hands hanging loosely by your sides.

2 Slowly bring your hips across to the left side, while moving your shoulders (keep them horizontal) to the right. This may be painful and cause twinges, and the muscles will tighten up in resistance. Maintain steady, relaxed breathing and sustain the stretch.

3 Relax and stand up straight, do not let your hips slip back to the right again. Repeat ten times, until you can return to a neutral position with no tilt.

4 Now perform a series of standing extension movements, see opposite.

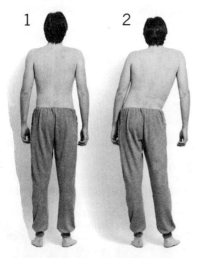

1   2

LOW BACK STRETCH

This is a very useful exercise if you have strained or dislodged a facet joint in your lower back and the surrounding muscles are tight and aching. It may also help if you are suffering from a recurrence of inflammation in worn facet joints, and it can improve flexibility if you have become stiff after an episode of acute low back pain. However, if your pain is caused by a disc protrusion, you may make it worse, so if the pain increases after two or three repetitions, do not continue with the exercise.

1 Lie down and do the basic pelvic tilt (see page 157).

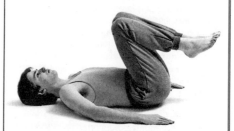

2 Keep your lower back flat and draw your knees up towards your chest.

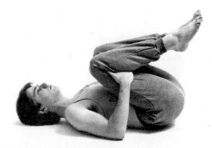

3 Grasp your legs behind your knees with both hands and squeeze your knees as close to your chest as possible. Breathe deeply. Maintain the squeeze for at least seven seconds.

4 Release your legs, lowering them slowly. Keep your knees bent and ensure that your back remains firmly pressed against the floor.

5 If your back arches as you lower your legs, you may feel a painful twinge, so try lowering one leg at a time.

STANDING EXTENSION

This gently arches your lower back, and should be performed every couple of hours throughout the day. If this exercise increases the pain in your back, it is still too soon after your acute attack started for you to do this exercise. Try the passive extension exercise instead, since this puts less strain on your back.

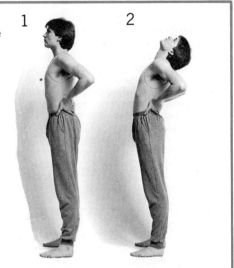

1 Stand up straight with your feet pointing directly forwards, about a shoulder width apart. Place your hands on the small of your back and breathe in deeply.

2 Breathe out slowly. As you do so, bend backwards, supporting your back with your hands, so that your lower back is arched. Repeat ten times.

MOBILIZING EXERCISES

These are generally useful for improving and maintaining mobility, which is of course essential to a healthy back. They can be helpful in most back conditions, with the usual proviso that you should stop at once if any of the exercises increases your pain. The mountain and sag exercise shown below, and the bending and twisting exercises overleaf gently stretch your muscles and prevent your spinal joints becoming stiff.

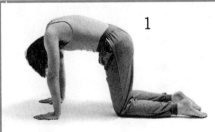

MOUNTAIN AND SAG

This consists of a series of rhythmic archings and roundings of the lower back. It is helpful in most cases of acute lower back pain, whether the pain is caused by facet joint or disc problems.

1 Start on your hands and knees, hunch your back like a cat and hold this position for about five seconds.

2 Gradually let your back sag down and hold for five seconds.

3 Hunch and sag your back alternately, starting gently and gradually increasing the range of movement.

4 If the extreme sag position is painful, allow your spine to drop to a point just before you know you are going to feel the twinge. Perform this exercise ten times every couple of hours during the day, until you can stand without pain.

GENTLE TWISTING

This is useful for improving general mobility, and particularly as an exercise for relaxing the muscles around the back and pelvic areas. It will also relieve pain caused by the facet joints by stretching the capsules and ligaments around the facet joints in the lower back: those on the left will be stretched as you drop your knees to the right, and vice versa.

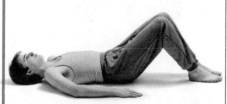

1 Lie on your back with your lower back pressed against the floor, your legs bent, your feet flat on the floor, and your arms by your sides, as for the pelvic tilt on page 157.

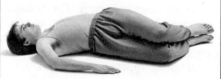

2 Keeping your knees together, let your legs flop slowly over to your right as far as they will go. Keep your left shoulder on the floor. Breathe slowly and deeply, and allow your legs and knees to drop a little further with each breath. Hold this position for a full minute, concentrating on relaxing rather than straining to achieve a goal.

3 Bring your knees back up and then lower them to the other side. Repeat the exercise, twisting to each side ten times.

SIDE BENDING

This exercise mobilizes the whole spine. The bending movements stretch the muscles around the waist and side of the trunk.

1 Stand with your feet a shoulder width apart and your arms by your sides.

2 Slide your right hand down the side of your right leg as far as you can and at the same time stretch your left arm up above your head. Keep the upper arm straight and as close as you can to the side of your head. Hold the stretch for at least seven seconds.

3 Slowly return to the upright position and lower your arm to your side. Repeat on the other side, then stretch down each side alternately a further nine times.

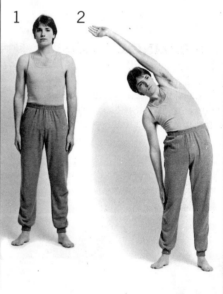

MUSCLE STRETCHING EXERCISES

Sometimes the mobility of the spine is restricted not just by stiffness in the joints and ligaments, but also because the muscles are not sufficiently flexible. People with chronic low back pain tend to develop tighter hamstring muscles, and sometimes even the calf muscles in the lower leg become tighter. In addition, inflexible leg muscles will make you prone to back trouble because you will tend to lift and bend in the wrong way, so these exercises, particularly the three hamstring stretches (opposite and overleaf), can be used preventatively.

CALF MUSCLE STRETCH

This increases the elasticity of the calf muscles and Achilles tendons at the back of the ankles.

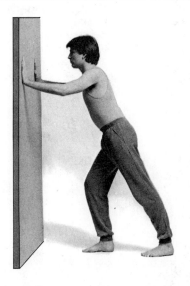

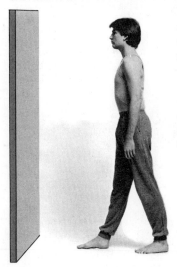

1 Stand facing a wall about an arm's length away, with your hands on the wall level with your shoulders. Point your feet straight towards the wall and keep your heels firmly on the ground throughout the exercise.

2 Bend your elbows and lean towards the wall, keeping your trunk and legs in a straight line. After a certain point you will feel a stretch in the back of the calf.

3 Hold this position for at least 15 seconds, then return to normal. Repeat ten times.

LYING HAMSTRING STRETCH

There are several ways in which to stretch the hamstring muscles, but some of them tend to pull on the joints of the lower back. This exercise does not put any excessive strain on your lower back, so if your back is at all painful or fragile, start with this hamstring exercise.

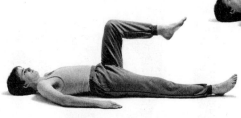

1 Lie on your back with your arms by your sides and your legs out straight. Raise your left leg, bending the knee to a right angle.

2 Slowly straighten your leg as much as you can, keeping the thigh vertical. Keep your right leg firmly on the floor. Hold the position for ten to 15 seconds to allow the muscle to relax and stretch.

3 Lower your leg slowly and repeat with your right leg. Repeat the exercise a further nine times on either side.

STANDING HAMSTRING STRETCH

This exercise will not strain your lower back. However, it requires some balance, so steady yourself by holding on to a piece of furniture when you first practise it. You may find this exercise easier if you hold your leg behind your knee to give it a little extra support.

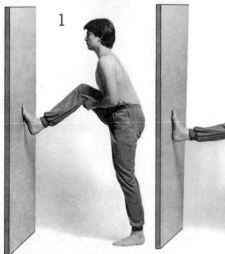

1 Stand facing a wall, a leg's length away. Raise your right leg with the knee bent, and place your foot at hip height on the wall. Keep your back and your left leg straight.

2 Slowly straighten your right leg, keeping the heel firmly against the wall. Maintain the stretched position for ten to 15 seconds. Repeat between six and ten times, then change legs.

THE LUMBAR PELVIC RHYTHM

This stretching exercise is more strenuous than the previous two hamstring stretching exercises, and you should not try it until your back is fairly strong and flexible. The aim is to master the lumbar pelvic rhythm. When you bend your back, your upper back should bend first, followed by the lower back, and finally the pelvis and hips. You should straighten up in reverse order. Some people automatically bend with this rhythm reversed, which puts excessive strain on the lower back, because half of the body passes well in front of the centre of gravity.

1 Stand with your feet together, and bend your neck until your chin touches your chest.

2 Slowly slide your hands down the front of your legs towards your knees, curling your back segment by segment, until your hands have reached as far as they will naturally go. Relax your neck and shoulders and keep your knees straight. Breathe freely and let your muscles go loose with each outward breath. Hang in this position for ten to 15 seconds, stretching out gently. Do not strain.

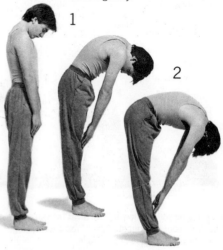

3 Return to the upright position in the reverse order: uncurl slowly and carefully from the hips first, then the lower back, segment by segment, until the neck and head straighten up. Make sure that your pelvis is tucked forwards, particularly as you unfold on the way up. Repeat this until you have mastered the rhythm.

THERAPEUTIC NECK EXERCISES

There are several exercises that can help you if you are prone to neck problems. Sometimes after poor posture has been sustained for a long time, the muscles will not relax at all and will ache continuously. This can cause quite severe pain, headaches, tingling and cold sensations around that area. If this is the case, the neck stretching exercise given overleaf may help, by encouraging your muscles to relax. It is particularly beneficial if you follow it up with a massage (see pages 172 to 173). Pain caused by discs or facet joints is more likely to be helped by passive extension of the neck, see below. The neck retraction exercise overleaf will help to relax your neck muscles, and if you practise it regularly, it should encourage you to hold your head correctly.

PASSIVE EXTENSION

The value of this exercise lies in allowing your head to provide traction for your neck. Do not attempt it if you are middle-aged or elderly and are prone to dizzy spells when you turn your head or look up.

1 Lie on your back on a flat couch or a firm bed with your shoulders on the edge, and your whole head, supported by your hands, projecting out over the end.

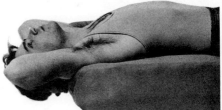

2 Still supporting your head on your hands, breathe out and let your head drop back very slowly and gently. Relax your neck muscles completely and let your hands support the full weight of your head.

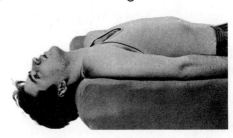

3 If you can allow your head to drop all the way back, your neck will be fully extended and you can take your hands away. Do not take your hands away if your head is not dropped right back. Remain in this position for about a minute initially, but after three or four attempts over the course of a day you should be able to stay like this for several minutes.

4 To get up after this, put your hands under your head and gently raise and support your head until your spine is straight. Roll over on to your stomach to stand up again.

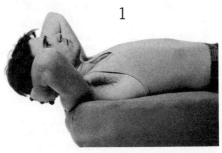

NECK RETRACTION

This will help to reduce postural pain. If practised regularly, it may prevent neck strain by encouraging better posture. Try it whenever you catch yourself holding your head forwards with your chin jutting out, for example, when you are driving a car, or leaning over a desk.

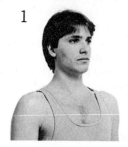
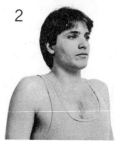
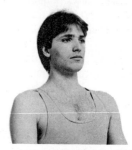

1 Look straight ahead and pull your chin back to straighten your neck. Make the crown of your head the highest point and elongate the distance between your shoulders and your ears.

2 Raise your shoulders, then lower them slowly while breathing out. Continue until your shoulders feel relaxed, keeping your neck straight and your chin pulled back.

NECK STRETCH

This exercise uses the weight of your head to stretch your neck muscles; it will reduce tension in your neck and shoulders. The instructions here start with stretching the left side — reverse them if you wish to stretch the right side first.

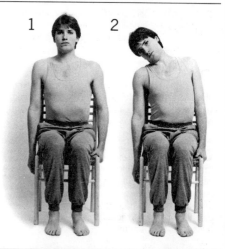

1 Sit down on an upright chair and hold the underside of the seat with your left hand.

2 Keep your left arm straight, and without raising your left shoulder, slowly lean your head and neck as far to the right as you can. Feel the stretch. Hold it for at least seven seconds and then return to the upright position. Repeat this several times on both sides, sustaining the stretch for as long as possible.

ANKYLOSING SPONDYLITIS

This inflammatory condition of the spine may affect other joints as well. As the disease progresses, the spine becomes increasingly bent forwards and restricted in all movements, particularly bending backwards. The joints where the ribs are attached to the vertebrae also become stiff, hampering chest expansion and breathing, and the hips also stiffen up. The exercises opposite and on page 166 are aimed at preventing this gradual stiffening process. Perform them every day, though not necessarily in this order.

NECK BEND

By encouraging you to hold your head properly, this exercise should help to prevent a stooped posture. Stand against a wall, push your head back towards the wall and hold it for a count of five, then relax. Repeat the exercise ten times.

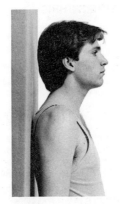 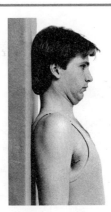

STANDING TWIST

Stand with your feet apart and place your hands on your hips. Turn from the waist to look behind you, then turn to the other side until you have twisted each way five times.

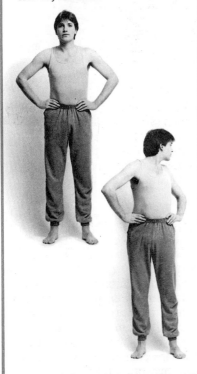

LEG AND SHOULDER RAISE

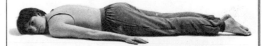

1 Lie on your front with your head turned to one side and your hands by your sides. Put a pillow under your chest if this allows you to lie more comfortably.

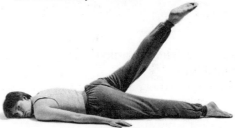

2 Keeping both legs straight, raise one leg as high as you can. Lower it again. Repeat five times for each leg.

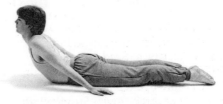

3 Raise your head and shoulders off the ground as high as you can. Repeat ten times.

DEEP BREATHING

1 Lie on your back with your knees bent and your feet flat on the ground. Put your hands on the ribs at the sides of your chest. Breathe in deeply through your nose and out through your mouth, pushing your ribs out against your hands as you breathe in. Repeat ten times.

2 Put your hands on the upper part of the front of your chest. Breathe in deeply through your nose and then breathe out as far as you can through your mouth. Try to push your ribs up against your hands as you breathe in. Breathe deeply in this way at least ten times.

ALTERNATE LIMB RAISE

Start on all fours, then stretch alternate arms and legs out parallel to the floor and hold for a count of ten. Lower and then repeat with the other arm and leg. Repeat five times each side.

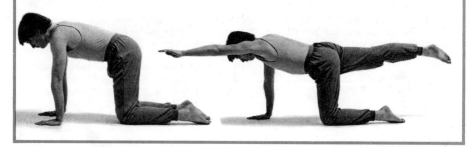

General advice for ankylosing spondylitis
● Lie on your front on a firm surface (with a pillow under your chest if necessary) for about 20 minutes every morning or evening.

● Repeat your deep breathing exercises at frequent intervals during the day.
● Beware of your posture; correct it constantly, not only during your exercise periods but during the day while standing, sitting and walking.

STRENGTHENING EXERCISES

As mentioned in earlier chapters, weak muscles, particularly weak abdominal muscles, may be a factor in causing back pain. Firm abdominal muscles improve posture by helping to keep the pelvis at the correct angle. Strong thigh muscles can prevent back trouble by allowing you to lift and bend correctly. Strong muscles in the back and neck themselves are probably of less value in preventing back pain, though as long as you are careful not to overstrain your back while you are exercising, strengthening these muscles may well be beneficial. You should not try any of these exercises while your back is hurting, but when the pain has subsided, these exercises may prevent a recurrence.

ABDOMINAL EXERCISES

A good way of developing the strength of your abdominal muscles is to practise the pelvic tilt, described on page 157. This can be done standing up, but lying down may be easier for a beginner.

The exercises given here are a useful way of supplementing the basic pelvic tilt and strengthening particular groups of abdominal muscles. The two below are isometric exercises, so-called because there is a maximum concentration of muscle power but a minimum change in length (*iso* = same; *meter* = length), so you hold certain muscles rigid while hardly moving that part of your body. The full sit-up is a more strenuous way of toning up these muscles.

HEAD AND SHOULDER RAISE

The head and shoulder raise is beneficial to all back conditions, and particularly suitable for people whose abdominal muscles are fairly weak and require further strengthening or for those who wish to trim excess weight off the abdomen. It is less strenuous than the full sit-up, but should not be tried while your back is hurting.

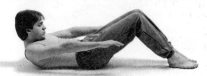

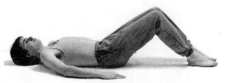

1 Lie on your back with your legs bent and the small of your back pressed against the floor, as for the pelvic tilt (see page 157).

2 Raise your head until your chin touches your chest, and reach forwards with your arms towards your lower leg on either side, raising your shoulders as high as you can off the floor. Make sure that your lower back remains firmly pressed against the floor.

3 Hold the raised position for a minimum of seven seconds and then release it slowly, uncurling from the back first, then the shoulders, and finally the neck. Repeat the exercise ten times in a session.

OBLIQUE ABDOMINAL EXERCISE

Another isometric exercise, this is particularly appropriate if you are keen on sports such as golf, which require turning movements of the trunk, and it is generally helpful for all back conditions, since it tones up the abdominal muscles. It is also useful for trimming weight off the sides of the abdomen and improving the waistline.

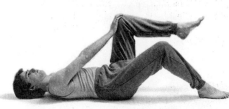

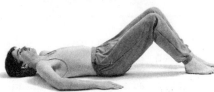

1 Lie down with your legs bent and your lower back pressed against the floor as for the basic pelvic tilt.

2 Raise your left knee up to a right angle, and reach with your right hand, keeping your arm straight, until it rests on the knee. Keep your lower back pressed against the floor.

3 Push as hard as possible with your arm and resist with your knee. Maintain this tension for at least seven seconds and then relax slowly, lowering your leg to the floor. Repeat, using your right leg and left arm. Perform the exercise a total of ten times on each side.

FULL SIT-UP

The full sit-up is another way of strengthening your abdominal muscles. Use it to keep yourself in good trim, and to prevent a recurrence of back trouble, but do not practise it when you are having an acute attack of back pain in case it is too strenuous. Always start this exercise with your legs bent, to avoid excessive strain on your lower back. If you are prone to recurring disc protrusion, be careful performing this exercise: stop at once if there is any pain, or seek advice from your therapist beforehand.

1 Lie down with the small of your back pressed against the floor and your knees bent.

2 Tuck your chin in towards your chest and reach forwards with your arms. Slowly straighten out your legs, to provide further leverage until you are sitting upright. Lean forwards to touch your toes, but do not overstrain.

3 Rest, take one breath in and let it out, then return in reverse order: bend your knees, keep your chin well tucked into your chest, your lower abdomen tight and your lower back rounded. Uncurl slowly from the base of the spine, controlling the movement all the way: do not flop or collapse.

4 Pause for at least one or two breaths before repeating this exercise. Repeat it ten times in one session initially. For greater fitness, do the exercise in sets of ten up to two or three times per exercise session.

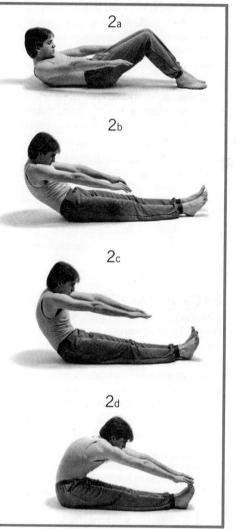

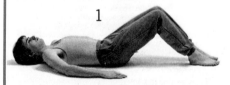

LEG EXERCISES

Strong reliable thigh muscles are important for lifting and bending. Unless you have knee problems, you should squat down, keeping your back straight and bending at the knees, when you reach for anything on the floor. Getting up from this position requires strong thigh muscles, and many people are not fit enough to rise up from their haunches even once, let alone repeatedly many times a day. It is no good trying to pick something up by bending your knees and keeping a straight back if you cannot get up again. When you first try this leg strengthening exercise (see Squats, opposite), make sure there is a table or a chair nearby to hold on to in case you cannot balance well enough. After a little practice, you will not need this.

SQUATS

You may find that you can manage only two or three repetitions at first, but do not worry: repeating this exercise two to three times a day over a few days will soon increase your strength until you can manage ten or even 20 repetitions with little effort.

1 Stand with your feet a shoulder width apart and tuck your pelvis in as for a standing pelvic tilt (see page 157).

2 Slowly bend at the knees holding on to nearby furniture if necessary, until you are squatting on your haunches. If you have arthritic knees, squat down as far as your knees allow.

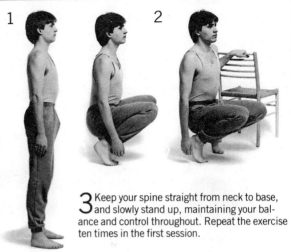

3 Keep your spine straight from neck to base, and slowly stand up, maintaining your balance and control throughout. Repeat the exercise ten times in the first session.

BACK EXERCISES

Contrary to popular belief, very few people have particularly weak back muscles; a so-called weak back is much more likely to be caused by some sort of defect in a spinal joint. On the whole, it is only manual workers, whose jobs entail lifting heavy weights regularly, who may need exercises to strengthen the back muscles after an injury or operation. Certain exercises have been prescribed for many years as a means of strengthening back muscles, but they tend to raise pressure in the discs and facet joints of the lower back, and often aggravate the condition.

HORIZONTAL RAISE

If you decide to try this exercise, do not raise your legs or shoulders above the horizontal, since this would increase the stress on your facet joints.

1 Lie face down across a firm chair or stool with your lower abdomen and pelvis supported. Make sure that you are well balanced so that your weight is evenly distributed on either side.

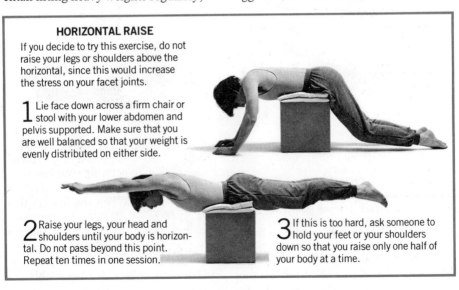

2 Raise your legs, your head and shoulders until your body is horizontal. Do not pass beyond this point. Repeat ten times in one session.

3 If this is too hard, ask someone to hold your feet or your shoulders down so that you raise only one half of your body at a time.

NECK EXERCISES

The three isometric exercises below are simple ways of strengthening your neck muscles by using your hands to prevent your head moving. Strengthening the muscles in the front of the neck is more awkward and not usually required since these muscles are very rarely weak. These are not relaxation exercises, and you should not do these exercises if your neck muscles are already very tense, as they could make your muscles feel even more tense. All three can be done either sitting or standing.

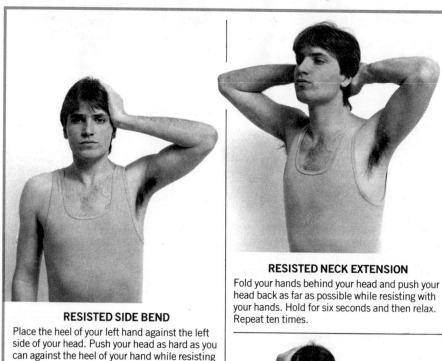

RESISTED NECK EXTENSION

Fold your hands behind your head and push your head back as far as possible while resisting with your hands. Hold for six seconds and then relax. Repeat ten times.

RESISTED SIDE BEND

Place the heel of your left hand against the left side of your head. Push your head as hard as you can against the heel of your hand while resisting with your arm. Do not move your head or your arm, but maintain maximum tension for at least six seconds. Repeat ten times, then repeat on the other side.

ROTATION

Place the heel of your right hand over your right temple and the heel of the left hand towards the back of your head on the other side. Try to turn your head towards the right, resisting with both arms. Hold for six seconds. Repeat ten times and then repeat the exercise, trying to the left.

SIMPLE RELAXATION

Muscle tension may be a response to a worrying or irritating situation, or to pain, or to postural stress. Whatever the reason for the tension, it can be a major cause of back and neck pain and one that you can often avoid if you teach yourself to recognize the danger signs and relax before it is too late.

Some muscle tension is, of course, essential for every move you make, but if you practise relaxation you will soon become aware of unnecessary tension in your body and learn how to release it. Before long you will notice when you are hunching your shoulders over the steering wheel while driving, or gripping the receiver too tight when telephoning. You will notice that you are sitting in a tense position during a meeting, or while feeding a baby. Whatever the demands on your life, you can learn to reduce the stress factor.

The simple exercises shown here make use of the principle that if you tighten one group of muscles the opposite group will relax. If you set aside a little time for them each day you will learn to release tension and relax fully, even if you are too busy for other, more strenuous exercises.

HOW TO RELAX

Remove your shoes and loosen any tight clothing. Listen to soothing music while you are doing this relaxation procedure, if this will help to reduce tension. Lie on your back on the floor or a firm bed with one pillow under your head, your arms by your sides or resting on your stomach, and your legs uncrossed. If your back aches or feels very tense, put a pillow under your knees. If your back is acutely painful or if you are heavily pregnant, you will probably find it more comfortable to lie on your side with your lower arm behind you, your upper knee bent forwards on a pillow and your lower leg straight. If you do not want to lie down at all, you can relax in an armchair, but make sure that your head and arms are fully supported and your legs are not crossed.

1 Start by pulling your shoulders down towards your feet. Lengthen the gap between your ears and your shoulders. Stop and feel the new position – it should be easy and comfortable.

2 Push your elbows out. Stop when your arms are comfortable and register this position.

3 Lengthen your fingers – stretch them to the fingertips and stretch your thumbs. Stop, and let them rest outstretched.

4 Tighten your buttocks and rotate your legs so your feet roll out. Let your legs feel heavy.

5 Move your knees around if you want to. Stop. Let your legs feel heavy again.

6 Push your feet gently down away from you. Stop and just let your feet hang comfortably off your ankles.

7 Press your body into the support behind you, if you are in a chair. Stop, then just let it sink into the support and enjoy this feeling.

8 Press your head back into the pillow or the back of the chair. Stop. Let the whole weight of your head sink into the pillow.

9 Close your eyes gently. Let your eyelids feel heavy. Open your mouth so that you un-clench your teeth. Close it gently. Push your tongue down on the bottom teeth, then let it rest in the middle of your mouth. Let your forehead feel smooth and comfortable, with no worry lines.

10 Be aware of your breathing. It will probably be slower now that you are relaxed. Be aware of taking air to the base of your lungs as you breathe in and then sigh out slowly. Continue breathing easily and comfortably while you rest for ten to 15 minutes, or for as long as you can.

RELAXATION THROUGH MASSAGE

This is another excellent way of relaxing tired and aching muscles and anyone can do it: contrary to popular belief, you do not need a full-scale course of instruction. In some parts of the world children learn to give and accept massage as part of their general upbringing. In the West, unfortunately, we seem to have lost contact with this traditional therapy, and have opted for more modern forms of healing. In spite of this, most people will admit that they would prefer a massage to a course of tranquilizers. Massage is also an ideal way of relieving backache during labour.

The general effect of a massage is to relax the muscles and to stimulate the circulation. The overall mental effect can be both relaxing and stimulating. A massage does not have to be extremely painful, but nor should it be absolutely painless. Particularly tense areas around the neck and shoulders may be trigger points, which are often painful when pressed firmly (see page 49). The tender areas should be massaged until they feel relaxed. If the muscle tightens or goes into spasm in response to pressure, then either the massage is too hard, or you are not able to tolerate that level of pain. Massage will help you identify areas of tension and this knowledge, as well as the massage itself, may help you to relax.

GIVING A MASSAGE

Choose a well-heated room and a firm, comfortable surface. Most beds are too soft, so it is generally better to lay a blanket or towel on the floor and ask your partner to lie down on his front.

Make sure that your hands are warm, and rub a little oil into the palms. Make and break contact gently, and massage with firm, rhythmic strokes, concentrating particularly on the tense areas.

MASSAGING THE BACK

The instructions below are for a complete back massage. If the person you are massaging suffers from aching muscles in just one region of the back, concentrate on that area. Unless otherwise specified, always work from the top of the spine downwards. Start strokes from the shoulders and work down to the mid back, or start at the mid back and work down from there to the buttocks.

1 Start with a few long, gentle strokes down the centre of the back from the base of the neck to the buttocks, and lightly up the sides.

2 Knead the shoulder muscles, gradually increasing the pressure. Work up the neck to the base of the skull.

3 Next, massage the shoulder blade area and the muscles around the mid spine using small circular movements, interspersed with longer, gentle strokes.

4 Apply thumb pressure down the bands of muscle by the spine, starting at the neck. When you reach the mid back, glide your hands up to the neck again and repeat. Follow with finger pressure on the same bands of muscle.

5 Apply hand pressure across the shoulders and right down the back to the buttocks.

6 Knead the large muscles of the lower back and buttocks.

7 Apply thumb pressure down the bands of muscle next to the spine from the mid back to the buttocks.

8 Work with circling movements on either side of the spine.

9 Apply hand pressure, starting at the mid back. Then, using the index and middle fingers of each hand, press firmly on the bands of muscles by the spine in short, overlapping strokes. Give firm strokes down the back with your hands flat, and finish the massage with long, soothing strokes.

BASIC TECHNIQUES

There are various strokes involved in giving a massage, appropriate to different stages of the massage, or to different areas of the body. These are some of the most useful for massaging the back; your partner will be able to tell you which are the most relaxing.

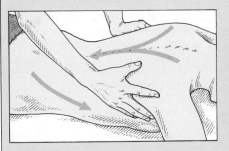

Long strokes
Gentle, sweeping strokes covering a wide area are a good way to start a massage. They spread the oil and prepare your partner for firmer strokes. Use your whole hand flat on the skin and make large circular movements. Start with very little pressure and gradually increase pressure.

Kneading
Squeeze the flesh gently between your fingers and thumbs in rippling movements, or between the heel of your hand and your fingers, as if kneading dough. This relaxes muscles, and should be used on fleshy areas such as shoulders, lower back and buttocks.

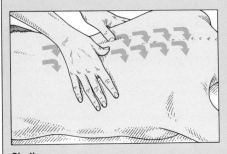

Circling
Press firmly, making circular movements. On small, tense areas, use just the tips of your fingers or your thumb. On wider or more fleshy areas, use the heel of your hand and work in much larger circles.

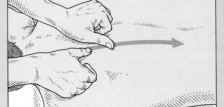

Thumb pressure
This is suitable for bands of tense muscle. Press firmly with your thumb in a long, smooth stroke.

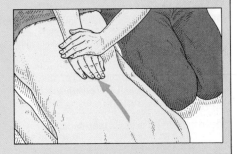

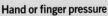

Hand or finger pressure
Place one hand flat on the skin, and the other hand on top. Press firmly and pull your hands along in short overlapping strokes. For smaller bands of muscle, make the same movement using the tips of your fingers.

ACUPRESSURE

This is a method of massage used to stimulate specific acupuncture points. It works on the same principle of stimulating points and meridians as acupuncture (see Chapter 11). The difference is that these points are stimulated by pressure, rather than with needles, so you can safely try this yourself without going to a specialist.

There are three main points for the relief of back pain and sciatica. Place the tip of one finger on the point indicated below. Press down hard and vibrate the finger rapidly but slightly for several minutes, or until the pain decreases. Relief from pain may last for only a few minutes, but sometimes it lasts for several days.

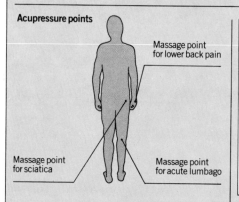

Acupressure points

Massage point for lower back pain

Massage point for sciatica

Massage point for acute lumbago

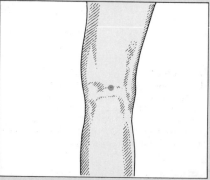

Acute lumbago

To relieve intense lower back pain which is restricting movement, press in the middle of the fold behind your knee on either leg.

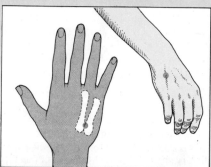

Lower back pain

Pain in the mid to lower back, particularly postural pain caused by prolonged sitting or standing may be relieved by pressure on this point.

Place your left forefinger between the knuckles of the ring finger and little finger on your right hand. Slide the finger down the back of your hand towards the wrist. You should be able to feel a slight dip between the bones leading to the knuckles. The acupressure point lies just where the bones meet, about two thirds of the way down from the knuckles to the wrist.

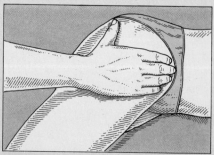

Sciatica

The point for relieving sciatica lies just behind the bony joint of the hip.

Lie down on your painless side with the affected leg half bent. Ask your partner to place his or her forefinger over the bony protrusion of the pelvis while keeping the thumb at right angles to the rest of the hand. The tip of the thumb will lie directly over the acupressure point.

15
Understanding and coping with pain

Most people with a physical cause of pain, such as back injury, also have a psychological component to their pain. Severe or prolonged pain results in dramatic changes of behaviour and mood, which in turn can affect the intensity of the pain. If you become depressed and worried by it, your pain will probably increase. Exaggerating your pain to others may also make it feel worse to you, but extreme stoicism is also unwise: it could make you very tense, and it might delay diagnosis and treatment.

You should not be alarmed if your doctor mentions that there is a psychological element in your pain, and you should not take this as a criticism. It is perfectly normal, and does not indicate any weakness in you. It does not mean that your pain is imaginary. If you have been in pain for months or years, your entire nervous system and personality will be affected. It is of enormous benefit to look at the problem of pain objectively, so that you can learn to minimize its effects and to live as full and enjoyable a life as possible.

Types of pain

The nature of your pain, as well as its severity, is an important clue to its cause. When you consult your doctor, your choice of words in describing the pain will help him to diagnose the problem (see page 75). Your descriptions may also tell you a good deal. It is quite possible that the words you use are influencing your own perception of the pain. If you regularly think about your pain as excruciating or unbearable, it may make the pain feel more intense. This applies only if you tend to use such terms loosely, and it does not imply that the pain is not excruciating sometimes.

PAIN PERCEPTION

The psychology of pain perception is only just beginning to be understood. The amount of pain you feel depends not only on the physical damage, but also on your mental state. It is possible to be unaware of some slight injury if your mind is occupied with something else. At the other extreme, there are numerous reports of people still feeling pain in an amputated limb. Clearly, there is an interaction between mental and physical factors in pain perception.

GATE CONTROL THEORY

Two renowned researchers in neuro-logy, Melzack and Wall, developed a model of pain perception to explain how these factors influence perception. Their theory is known as the Gate Control Theory, because they visualized these factors opening or closing a gate, there-by stimulating or inhibiting the amount of pain that is felt.

Normally the gate is closed and no pain is felt. It is only when a part of the body is damaged that the various factors start battling to push the gate open or to close it again. The intensity of pain depends on how wide open the gate is.

Neural impulses

The gate is pushed open by nerves known as S-fibres (small fibres), which relay messages of pain from the site of injury or inflammation. Longer fibres (L-fibres) are stimulated by massage, aromatic rubs and other therapies, and help to close the gate, reducing the intensity of the pain message.

When the gate is opened – which hap-pens if the impulses from the S-fibres swamp those from the L-fibres – a cell known as the T-cell is triggered, and pain messages are relayed through the nervous system towards the brain. But this does not necessarily mean that you will feel any pain. The neural impulse passes through the brain stem in the neck, to the centre of the brain, and then to the outer cortex of the brain, where it is finally translated into a con-scious perception of pain. At any of these stages in its journey, the pain message can be blocked.

Arousal system activity

Some functions of the nervous system are controlled from a centre in the brain stem, and are known collectively as the arousal system. When this system is active, pain messages are muted before they reach the brain. The arousal sys-tem is less active when the brain is highly active, for example, when you are worried or frightened, and it can

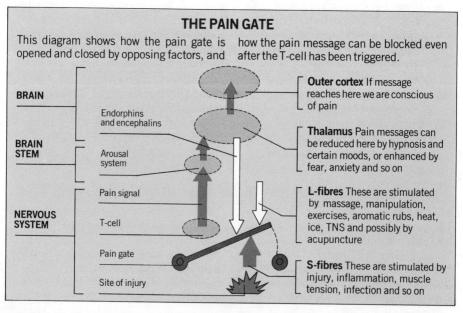

THE PAIN GATE

This diagram shows how the pain gate is opened and closed by opposing factors, and how the pain message can be blocked even after the T-cell has been triggered.

BRAIN

BRAIN STEM

NERVOUS SYSTEM

Endorphins and encephalins

Arousal system

Pain signal

T-cell

Pain gate

Site of injury

Outer cortex If message reaches here we are conscious of pain

Thalamus Pain messages can be reduced here by hypnosis and certain moods, or enhanced by fear, anxiety and so on

L-fibres These are stimulated by massage, manipulation, exercises, aromatic rubs, heat, ice, TNS and possibly by acupuncture

S-fibres These are stimulated by injury, inflammation, muscle tension, infection and so on

FACTORS AFFECTING PAIN PERCEPTION

Susceptibility to pain is greater when the brain is highly active or when the arousal system is inactive. Decreased brain activity and increased arousal system activity both dull the intensity of pain. The mental and physical states listed below influence pain perception, either exaggerating or dulling the intensity of pain.

Decrease pain	Increase pain
■ Emotional tranquillity	■ Anxiety and uncertainty
■ Sleep	■ Fear
■ Hypnosis	■ Depression
■ Hyperventilation (which causes reduced carbon dioxide)	■ Concentrating attention on pain
■ Excess alcohol	■ Drinking small amounts of tea, coffee and alcohol
■ Distracting attention from your pain	■ Drugs such as marijuana, LSD and barbiturates
■ Increase in adrenalin	
■ Drugs such as valium and morphine	

also be made less active by drugs such as barbiturates. In these states, then, you will feel more intense pain. The arousal system is active when your mind is calm, when you are asleep or under hypnosis, and when you take certain drugs such as valium or morphine. All of these factors reduce the amount of pain you feel.

Pain-reducing hormones

The brain itself can also close the pain gate. As the message reaches the brain, before you consciously feel any pain, the brain stimulates the production of pain-reducing hormones, encephalins and endorphins (the body's own version of morphine). These help to reduce your perception of pain.

Drugs such as morphine and valium can supplement your own endorphins, in order to enhance the pain-reducing effect. There is some evidence that acupuncture controls pain by stimulating the production of endorphins, and it may also stimulate L-fibres directly.

MENTAL ATTITUDES

Pain messages can also be blocked or reduced between the centre of the brain and the outer cortex, which translates the message into a conscious feeling of pain. Your general state of mind – including your will to recover, your expectations and anxieties, your mood and your ability to concentrate on something else – is the decisive factor here. Pain control therapies such as hypnosis, and the placebo effect (that is, many people benefit as much from fake pain-killers as from real ones, provided they believe that they have taken real drugs), probably block messages at this stage. The mind, in effect, has an arsenal of weapons, conscious and subconscious, which can work to subdue or to increase the level of pain

Motivation

Just as the brain is capable of limiting the amount of pain you feel, so it can exaggerate the pain and delay recovery. Inevitably, not everyone is equally motivated to recover quickly from a back problem. Some people have an enjoyable social life and a rewarding job: they will be keen to return to normal life, and this will speed up their recovery. Others are stuck on a treadmill. They will probably welcome the extra attention and sympathy they get from being ill, and there may be other rewards, such as a good sick pay scheme or industrial compensation. These people are likely to take longer to recover, though they will be totally unconscious of wanting to remain ill. Their recovery might be speeded up by measures apparently unrelated to their back condition, such as changing jobs or taking on different duties at work. If you feel reluctant to return to work after a lengthy illness, it is probably worth asking your employer if you could change the nature of your work, or asking your doctor to make this request on your behalf.

Emotional reactions to pain

Pain and depression are very closely linked: pain will make you depressed, and depression will make you more susceptible to pain. It is likely that most people in chronic pain feel depressed.

Surveys show that about half of all patients with psychiatric illness also have physical pain, and roughly half of these complain of back pain. Feelings of anxiety are another common result of long-term pain. Learning how to overcome both depression and anxiety is an important part of coping with chronic pain. Some advice is given on page 181.

Personality and pain

Research in North America on chronic pain has identified two particular personality traits, hysteria, and hypochondriasis, which are common among those people whose pain does not decrease following lengthy conservative treatment. The terms in this context have a slightly different meaning from their normal usage. Hysteria indicates someone who has a variety of physical symptoms, and who is also dissatisfied with life and generally unhappy. Hypochondriasis describes someone with a wide range of physical complaints involving several different functions of the body.

As well as identifying which types of people do not respond to therapy, it is possible to establish certain types of personality or background which make people more prone to feeling pain. These traits include:
- Feelings of guilt
- A strong, unfulfilled aggressive drive
- Pain developing after loss – such as bereavement or divorce – or after threatened loss
- Inactivity, inability to enjoy social life, leisure or sex, and lack of initiative
- Denial of conflicts
- A history of suffering, defeat and a fear of success
- Depression or alcoholism in the family, or a relative in chronic pain.

The effect on others

Your pain may also affect the mood and behaviour of people around you, in much the same way as it affects you. If you have been in pain for some time and those caring for you at home become irritable, it is important to recognize that these changes in behaviour are a by-product of your illness. People caring for you are probably just as worried and depressed by your pain as you are. Anyone who is caring for a patient in chronic pain must try to strike a balance between being over-attentive and fussy (which will encourage you to concentrate on your pain) and being impatient and off-hand (which might make you resentful and depressed). The best way of caring for someone in chronic pain is to encourage normal activity and independence as much as possible, while remaining sympathetic and making allowances for your pain and disability.

Remember that the way in which you describe pain may affect other people's reactions. If you are very stoical and refuse to acknowledge any pain, other people may think you are moody when you are simply suppressing your reaction to pain. On the other hand, if you tend to dramatize or overstate your pain, you may irritate and bore other people, rather than arousing their sympathy.

Your disability may have a serious effect on your partner's life, particularly if he or she is having to carry you, or help you with basic activities such as feeding, washing or dressing. It is worth while exploring your reactions to the new situation, and you should discuss this together. The extra work thrown on to your partner by your disability may be making you feel guilty and your partner feel resentful.

COPING WITH PAIN

We are not, on the whole, brought up to cope with pain as a way of life; most people with long-term back pain are experiencing a whole range of emotional and psychological problems which they have not previously encountered and which they are not trained to handle. To consult a professional, whether a psychologist or other therapist, is to tackle your problem in a practical manner: it is a sign of strength not of weakness.

If your back condition is unlikely to improve with further treatment, for example if spinal surgery has failed, you should seek help for coping with long-term pain. However, it is essential that - you have realistic expectations when you start any course of treatment. This way, you will avoid disappointment and a sense of failure. If your pain will not disappear, you should aim to diminish its impact on your life, and to find ways of decreasing the pain itself. It is important to remember that therapies to help you cope with pain can succeed only if you participate actively in them.

Many of the techniques discussed here will teach you ways of helping yourself. You can learn to change self-defeating patterns of thought and behaviour, and to adapt to a new lifestyle.

The best way to start is to become aware of how your mood can affect your pain. Think how a small child makes a big fuss about a slight graze, if he knows he will get attention, but will forget all about it as soon as he sees the ice-cream van. The starting point for pain therapy is recognizing such behaviour in yourself, and cultivating distractions.

RELAXATION

Learning a relaxation technique will reduce your pain by giving you greater conscious control over your own body. It will make you aware of tension and stress and enable you to relax mentally and to release particular muscles, which may have tensed up in response to pain. Relaxation also influences the arousal system (see page 176), and this may underlie the feeling of improvement.

EMG feedback

One method of relaxation training uses EMG (electromyographic) feedback, which gives you clear information about the tension in your muscles. Sensors are placed on particular groups of muscles, usually around the neck and shoulder area or on the lower back. They are attached to a small machine which gives off a signal – a click or a flashing light. The tenser the muscles, the faster the signal emitted by the machine.

Your doctor will refer you to a special clinic or perhaps to a physiotherapist for the treatment. Your first sessions using

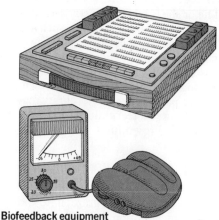

Biofeedback equipment
Several types of machines are available that can feed back information about various body functions such as brain-wave patterns and electrical skin resistance, as well as muscle tension.

an EMG machine will be with a therapist, and you will be lying down to start with. Later on, you can use the machine while sitting, standing or walking. If you want to use the machine at home, your therapist may be able to advise you where to buy one.

To use the equipment, sit or lie comfortably, and concentrate on slowing the signal down. Some people benefit considerably from such direct feedback, and learn quickly how to relax their muscles. Unfortunately, though, there is no consistent relationship between the EMG change and the subjective change.

Studies have shown that after only ten sessions, most patients feel much less pain; they need, on average, only half the amount of pain-killers and have become much more active.

Other relaxation methods

There are a number of ways to achieve deep muscle relaxation without the aid of an EMG feedback machine. These include autogenic training, contract-relax, and meditation. You can learn any of these techniques from a trained

therapist or from tape-recorded lessons, and then practise them on your own.

The autogenic approach is a form of autosuggestion or self-hypnosis (see page 129), in which you repeat certain phrases instructing various muscle areas to relax. The repetition of these verbal cues can enable you to relax quickly and at will if you practise regularly.

The contract-relax technique is similar to the simple relaxation technique on page 171. It encourages you to recognize the difference between tensing your muscles briefly but strongly, and then relaxing them completely. The sudden change from one extreme to the other enhances awareness of the amount of tension in your muscles. Meditation can also reduce tension. See page 130 for a simple meditation technique.

In some respects the EMG machine provides a short-cut to all these more traditional methods by providing you automatically with information about the tension in your body. If you have been in chronic pain for several months, you may not be aware how tense your muscles have become, so the direct feedback from an EMG machine could be useful before you practise any of the other methods given here.

The success of these methods is influenced greatly by the result of the initial session. For example, if pain has disturbed your sleep for several days and you sleep soundly after the first relaxation session, subsequent sessions are likely to be successful, too. In addition, if you keep a record of the level of pain you experience before and after relaxation sessions, any improvement can be noted, and will encourage you to continue with the technique.

Staying relaxed

When you can relax at will, try to apply the techniques throughout the day. A visual cue might help to remind you – mark a cross on a small card and stick this to your bedroom mirror, on your office desk, above the kitchen work top, next to your rear view mirror in the car or even over the head of your bed. As soon as you catch sight of this cue, adopt the particular technique that you have learned until you feel more relaxed. With time and practice, this can become automatic, so that you are in a natural state of relaxation.

TACKLING YOUR MOOD

Certain moods, particularly depression and anxiety, can heighten sensitivity to pain and delay recovery. Both can be caused by chronic pain in the first place, so a vicious circle can easily develop. It is therefore extremely important to recognize these moods in yourself, and to try to overcome them.

Depression

As a medical term, depression means more than simple unhappiness; it includes a number of physical changes as well. If you have most or all of the following symptoms, you should seek help for depression:
● reduced or greatly increased appetite and weight
● marked changes of mood
● lethargy and listlessness
● inability to enjoy any pastime
● disturbed sleep.

One way to minimize or prevent depression is to focus on the clear physical source of your pain, but doctors and other practitioners often prescribe drugs to treat depression. The drugs most commonly used are called "tricyclics". It may be two or three weeks before you notice any effect, but you should always follow your doctor's instructions precisely and take the full course of drugs. Tricyclics are not addictive, but they

may make you feel drowsy. While taking these drugs you may also find that your heart races and your mouth is dry, you might have difficulty passing urine and your vision might become blurred. Other anti-depressant drugs are extremely effective, but some have to be given under strict supervision because they react badly with certain foods and drinks and other drugs.

Anxiety

People in chronic pain often become very anxious, without necessarily having a definite cause for their worry. Tranquillizers such as valium can calm you down, especially if you are worrying about something specific, such as an operation. However, these drugs cannot be used over a long time since they are addictive and do not help you to overcome your anxiety. Never harbour any hidden fears about your illness, since this will add to your stress; always discuss them with your doctor.

Some people experience severe panic attacks, which are isolated episodes approaching extreme terror, accompanied by a variety of physical symptoms such as palpitations, pains in the chest, shortness of breath, and panting. A few even develop phobias such as agoraphobia – the fear of going into open public places. Naturally, these complications are severely disabling, both for the individual and the surrounding family. Some drugs, such as Imipramine (one of the tricyclic anti-depressants) can block or prevent the occurrence of these panic attacks.

REDUCING PAIN BEHAVIOUR

People who are in pain for several months or years often undergo significant changes in their general behaviour and personality. They learn that they will win sympathy from those around them, and will be offered pain-killers, as soon as they show their discomfort by groaning or complaining. They become conditioned to complain about even the slightest twinge, and this type of behaviour itself delays their return to active and enjoyable life.

Pain clinics

Special clinics have been set up to reverse the conditioning process that leads to this pattern of behaviour. Some of these clinics admit patients for several weeks, others take day patients. Staff at the clinics give attention and praise to those who do not complain and who try to keep active, while ignoring patients when they complain. Since many of the patients complain about their pain in order to be given pain-killers, these drugs are administered under strict supervision at fixed intervals, regardless of the patient's behaviour. The pain-killers are given in a strongly flavoured drink, so that the dose can be reduced without the patient becoming aware of it – all must agree to this procedure before they are admitted to the clinic.

After a few weeks of this treatment your pain should feel much less severe. You will be more cheerful as you will be able to take part in everyday activities, and consequently you will find that you do not complain about the pain as much as you used to.

Adaptive response training

For some people, pain can become a protective shell behind which it is easy to retreat when life becomes too hard to handle. It provides the ideal excuse for getting out of any unpleasant chores or activities. Such people exaggerate the pain to themselves and to others, in order to avoid certain situations, until the pain becomes a necessary part of their lives. Shy people may use back

pain as an excuse for avoiding social occasions. Others may use it to get out of housework or even to avoid sex.

Your doctor will refer you to a specialist if he feels that this therapy is appropriate. Adaptive response training teaches people to examine themselves critically to discover whether they are using back pain as an excuse in certain situations. They are then encouraged to tackle problems, such as shyness or family difficulties, head on, so that they no longer need the excuse of back pain.

Defeating insomnia

Adaptive response training can also be used to help cure the insomnia which plagues many people with chronic back pain. The therapy encourages you to tackle your sleep problem head on, instead of letting your pain rule your sleeping habits. It aims to establish routines conducive to a normal sleep pattern. The basic instructions include:
● Only lie down to sleep when you are feeling sleepy.
● Do not do anything (apart from sexual activity) in bed except sleep.
● If you do not fall asleep within 15 minutes of getting into bed, get up and leave the bedroom. Do not return to bed until you are sleepy.
● Set the alarm for the same time every morning, and get up regardless of how much sleep you have had.
● Avoid day time naps.
● Avoid coffee, tea and other stimulants, which may exacerbate insomnia.

Stress inoculation therapy

Like the other therapies discussed in this section, stress inoculation therapy aims to alter patients' attitudes to their pain. It works well for people with chronic headaches, but has not yet been fully assessed as a treatment for chronic back pain. The therapy is given in groups by a physiotherapist. Sufferers are encouraged to examine in detail the nature of their pain and its effect on their lives. They are given a full explanation of the nature of their disorder, and are taught special techniques for coping with individual aspects of the pain, for example, ways of changing position from sitting to standing to avoid sharp twinges.

NEURO-STIMULATION

Over 2,000 years ago a Roman writer reported that pain in the feet due to such problems as gouty arthritis could be relieved by placing the feet in a bucket of water along with an electric eel. This delivered an electric shock which banished pain for some hours.

The idea may sound strange, but the principle does work, though exactly why is not known. Electrical stimulation probably reduces pain partly by stimulating the L-fibres which close the pain gate (see page 176) and interrupt the pain messages from S-fibres. It also increases the level of the body's pain-inhibiting hormones, the endorphins and encephalins, which circulate in the cerebro-spinal fluid bathing the nerves in the spinal canal.

Many pain clinics all over the world now offer neuro-stimulation to alleviate both acute and chronic pain.

Transcutaneous stimulation

This treatment is the most common method of stimulating nerves electrically. You will probably be treated in a physiotherapy department. Electrodes will be placed on your skin in carefully selected positions, most probably at one of the following sets of points:
● tender trigger points in the painful region
● distant trigger points (if no local ones are found)
● major peripheral nerves associated with the painful area
● acupuncture points (there are acupuncture points for various pain patterns and they often overlap with trigger points, which in turn tend to lie over major sensory nerves).

A low voltage current is passed through the electrodes and increased until you find the sensation slightly painful, and the level is then adjusted to

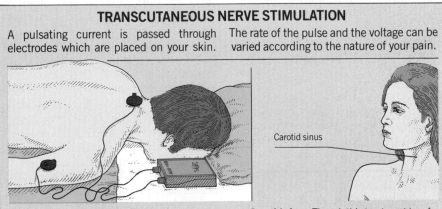

TRANSCUTANEOUS NERVE STIMULATION

A pulsating current is passed through electrodes which are placed on your skin.

The rate of the pulse and the voltage can be varied according to the nature of your pain.

Carotid sinus

Treatment session You may need to lie down for your first session, but later on you can use the equipment standing up or moving around.

Carotid sinus Though this treatment is safe enough to be used at home, never place the electrodes over the carotid sinus in your neck.

just below this threshold. Provided the pain is relieved, the treatment will last about 20 minutes and you will probably have between three and five sessions a week, until your pain is reduced semi-permanently. Once you can use the stimulator yourself, you may be able to borrow one for use at home.

The method is quite safe, though there are certain restrictions for people with cardiac pacemakers or who are in the first three months of pregnancy.

About 60 per cent of patients find that this treatment reduces their pain. Some have rather short-lived relief, but about 50 per cent experience continuing bene fit from six to 18 months after their treatment has ended.

One of the advantages in this treatment is that it makes analgesics and narcotics redundant. These drugs may be very effective in dealing with acute pain, but if used on a long-term basis they suppress the body's ability to produce its own natural analgesics, the endorphins and encephalins.

Implanted neuro-stimulators

If the pain is severe enough, nerves can be stimulated by implanting a stimulator at the back of the spinal cord. This can be very effective but it is much less common than TNS treatment, and is restricted to use in cases where back surgery has failed. It is particularly useful for people whose nerves have been irreparably damaged.

Under a local anaesthetic, tiny electrodes are placed in the epidural space, usually about half way down the back. Leads will run under your skin, coming out at the sides to connect to a minute generator, which you will be able to operate manually to test the system. If it gives you sufficient pain relief, the entire system can be put under the skin in a second operation. The stimulator is

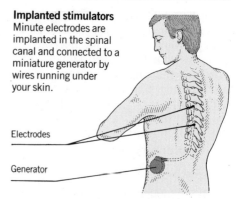

Implanted stimulators
Minute electrodes are implanted in the spinal canal and connected to a miniature generator by wires running under your skin.

Electrodes

Generator

powered by batteries which should last for five years and can be replaced in a minor operation. Stimulation can be altered by a radio-controlled external programmer, and you can turn the system on and off using a magnet.

Between 50 and 60 per cent of users benefit from an epidural nerve stimulation system. It is best used intermittently rather than continuously, because this increases the body's production of natural pain-reducing hormones.

The pain is not completely relieved by this implant, and you will still feel any sharply localized pain. As with other electrical nerve stimulation treatment, the implant blocks pain by stimulating the L-fibres which close the pain gate (see page 176). It has the further advantage of increasing the blood flow to a formerly painful extremity by dilating the blood vessels. This is particularly helpful for the diffuse burning pain caused by damage to the sympathetic nerves. An implant can even heal ulcers caused by poor circulation.

People who remain on narcotic medicines after an implant often feel the electrical sensation of stimulation, but obtain no pain-relief from it. Their pain can be reduced by taking certain nutritional supplements and anti-depressant drugs, which increase production of the body's own pain-reducing hormones.

Deep brain stimulators

A tiny minority of people with very severe and widespread pain are treated with a neuro-stimulator implanted in the brain. The stimulating electrode is placed deep in the brain, in the grey matter surrounding one of the chambers, or in one of the nuclei of the thalamus (the central structure which receives pain messages). Since there is a slight risk of brain damage, this operation is done only in extreme cases.

While spinal stimulators work by closing the pain gate and blocking the pain messages before they reach the brain, the deep brain stimulators appear to encourage production of the body's own pain-reducing hormones.

At present research is underway with the aim of developing new devices that will function automatically according to the body's needs. The system will switch on and off according to the levels of hormones circulating in the body.

A SENSE OF SELF-CONTROL

People with chronic back pain may develop a sense of disappointment and failure, which can lead to despair. You can avoid this by initiating short-term constructive goals, but do not have unrealistic expectations. Set yourself a daily target, so that you can achieve something every day. It is much better to have a specific aim, like walking one kilometre (half a mile) *this* morning, rather than a general target such as recovering by the end of the summer. Your therapist might be able to help by setting specific short-term goals such as weight loss, and by developing an exercise programme. Keep a daily record of your progress so that you will feel a sense of achievement, rather than just brooding on your symptoms and your disability. When you feel more self-confident, you may be able to take up a

sport, but you should ask your therapist for advice on which sports are suitable for your back condition.

Living with pain

If your pain is persistent, it is inadvisable to use drugs continually. You must try to control the pain yourself, and learn to live with it. Some of the techniques suggested here may help to reduce your pain, but the most important element is your mental attitude.

Avoid concentrating on your pain: focus your attention on other things, and take up interests that will not harm your back or aggravate your pain. Try not to drop out of social occasions; if you have to stay in bed for a long time, invite close friends to visit you. If you notice a change in your relationship with your partner, consider whether it is due to your back condition. Always discuss any such problems together – chronic pain in one partner puts a strain on both, so you must try to understand each other's reaction to the situation.

Return to your normal activities as far as possible, though you will have to make allowances for your back. Adapt your home to avoid putting unnecessary strain on your back – follow the advice given in Chapter 13. If you have a sedentary job, try to use a chair which will support your spine, adjust the height of your work surface if possible, and store things at easily accessible heights. If you have a manual job, pay special attention to your back when you lift and carry anything, and stay off work if your pain flares up. You may find that exercises help to control the pain and prevent you getting tense.

So long as you maintain a positive attitude, and do not let the pain control your life, you will almost certainly be able to return to most of your normal activities, and lead a full and active life.

Conclusion

Although backache is an enormous problem, it is one that could in part be solved. We already know enough to prevent much disability from back pain. The problem is that this knowledge is not applied, and many useful therapies are not readily available. If the proposals below were implemented, which is no mean task I will fully admit, I estimate that prolonged disability due to back trouble could be reduced by at least 70 per cent.

● All medical students and physiotherapists should receive adequate training in orthopaedic medicine.
● All general practitioners, orthopaedic surgeons, rheumatologists and physical medicine specialists should learn manipulative and injection techniques for treating musculo-skeletal disorders.
● All physiotherapists should learn techniques of manipulative medicine and when to apply them.
● All "alternative" practitioners who hold a degree in osteopathy, chiropractic, or acupuncture from a recognized training college, should be accepted into the nation's existing health service, to treat musculo-skeletal disorders.
● All patients should have early access to one of the above professionals to receive appropriate advice and treatment.

While there is much that the medical profession can do, many of the answers lie with the individual. Poor posture and careless use of the back are among the most common causes of back trouble. The adverse effects of our increasingly sedentary way of life could be minimized through improved education. Children should be made aware of the importance of good posture, and adults should keep fit by exercising and taking part in sports.

Chapter 13 offers advice and instructions on how to reduce stress on your spine as you go about your everyday activities. However, these instructions apply only to isolated moments, removed from the general flow of actions. They should be complemented with awareness of your posture, how tense you are, and where you feel tense.

Central to this self-awareness is correct breathing. Notice how often in a day you are holding your breath or breathing quickly and shallowly at a tense moment. Whenever you catch yourself breathing like this, pause and focus your attention on your breathing. You will soon be able to regain a steady, relaxed rhythm of breathing without any tension in the upper abdomen. Steady, relaxed breathing is essential for fluent, coordinated and efficient movement. You will also benefit from the mental effect of relaxation – reduced anxiety.

This freedom from anxiety has a part to play in the prevention of back pain. Mental stress and physical tension almost invariably go together. Thus the second step in the prevention of back trouble is to reduce muscular tension by avoiding stressful situations or learning to cope with them. Acute back and neck problems may indicate that your body can no longer tolerate your lifestyle. If you have back pain, it may be useful to regard it as your body's warning sign.

Finally, remember that there are many different therapies for treating back trouble, and if your own self-help measures are not enough, search around until you find one that works for you.

Useful addresses

GENERAL HEALTH

Health Education Council
78 New Oxford Street
London WC1A 1AH
01-637 1881
(general information service, publishes leaflets)

Age Concern
Bernard Sunley House
60 Pitcairn Road
Mitcham, Surrey
01-640 5431
(national centre for 950 independent groups serving the needs of elderly people)

Royal Association for Disability and Rehabilitation
25 Mortimer Street
London W1N 8AB
01-637 5400
(publishes information, offers advice on social and legal aspects of disability)

Intractable Pain Society of Great Britain and Ireland
Basingstoke District Hospital
Aldermaston Road
Basingstoke
Hants RG24 9NA
0256 473202
(has a register of all pain clinics in Britain)

BACK PAIN

Back Pain Association
31-33 Park Road
Teddington
Middlesex TW11 0AB
01-977 5474/5

(supports research into back disorders, publishes information on causes and prevention of back pain)

ANKYLOSING SPONDYLITIS

National Ankylosing Spondylitis Society
6 Grosvenor Crescent
London SW1X 7ER
01-637 5400
(for free information booklet, counselling service, branches throughout the country for group therapy)

ARTHRITIS

Arthritic Association
44 Glenville Road
Walkford
Christchurch
Dorset
04252 3106

Arthritis and Rheumatism Council
41 Eagle Street
London WC1R 4AR
(sponsors research and publishes information)

COMPLEMENTARY MEDICINE

British Holistic Medical Association
179 Gloucester Place
London NW1
01-262 5299
(publishes information)

Institute for Complementary Medicine
21 Portland Place
London W1N 3AS
01-636 9543
(publishes information)

ACUPUNCTURE

British Acupuncture Association
34 Alderney Street
London SW1V 4EM
01-834 1012/834 3350
(publishes a register of members)

Council for Acupuncture
10 Belgrave Square
London SW1X 8PH
(publishes a list of all British acupuncturists registered with three main acupuncture organizations)

MANIPULATIVE THERAPIES

The General Council and Register of Osteopaths
1-4 Suffolk Street
London SW1Y 4HG
01-839 2060
(publishes a register of about 850 professionally qualified osteopaths, supplies names of local practitioners)

Institute of Orthopaedic Medicine
30 Park Row
Nottingham NG1 6GR
0602 411544

The Society of Orthopaedic Medicine
19 Jesmond Road
Hove BN3 5LN
0273 410826
(runs courses for doctors and physiotherapists, provides list of local therapists)

British Chiropractic Association
5 First Avenue
Chelmsford
Essex CM1 1RX
0245 353078/358487
(publishes information leaflets and supplies a list of local practitioners)

Manipulation Association of Physiotherapists
c/o Honorary Secretary
Mrs A Middleditch
55 Hamilton Road
Thornton Heath
Surrey CR4 8NN

Society of Teachers of the Alexander Technique
10 London House
266 Fulham Road
London SW10 9EL
01-351 0828
(send a stamped addressed envelope for information and a list of local teachers)

HOMEOPATHY

The British Homeopathy Association
27a Devonshire Street
London W1N 1RJ
01-935 2163
(can supply a list of practitioners and pharmacists, holds lectures, publishes information and has a library for members)

The Royal London Homeopathic Hospital
Great Ormond Street
London WC1
01-837 3091
(NHS hospital specializing in homeopathic treatment. Send a stamped addressed envelope for information and a list of NHS and private homeopathic doctors)

HYPNOTHERAPY

National Register of Hypnotherapists and Psychotherapists
National College of Hypnotists and Psychotherapists
25 Market Square
Nelson
Lancs
0282 699378
(can supply a list of qualified practitioners)

British Society of Medical and Dental Hypnosis
42 Links Road
Ashtead
Surrey KT21 2HJ
03722 73522
(runs courses for doctors and dentists, publishes a register of members and supplies a list of local practitioners)

Centre for Autogenic Training
Positive Health Centre
101 Harley Street
London W1
01-935 1811
(offers group and individual training)

MEDITATION

Transcendental Meditation Center
Roydon Hall
7 Mile Lane
Tunbridge, Kent
0622 813243

KEEPING FIT

The Sports Council
16 Upper Woburn Place
London WC1H 0QP
01-388 1277

Scotland
031-225 8411

Wales
0222 397571

(Sports Councils have lists of sports centres in England, Wales and Scotland and publish brochures of courses)

EQUIPMENT

Equipment for the Disabled
Mary Marlborough Lodge
Nuffield Orthopaedic Centre
Headington
Oxford
0865 750103
(publishes information on aids to help the disabled)

Backswing (UK) Ltd
Lecton House
Lake Street
Leighton Buzzard
Bedfordshire
0525 383100
(direct mail order for inversion therapy equipment and Balans chair)

Index

Page numbers in *italic* refer to illustrations and captions

A

abdominal exercises, *167-8*
abscesses, 63, 64
acupressure, 125-6, *174*
acupuncture, 39, 40, 42, 50, 60-1, 62, 118-26, *119*, *123-5*
  conditions that may respond, 121
  consulting an acupuncturist, 121-5
  electronic acupuncture, 126, *126*
  meridians, 118-19, *119*
  pain relief, 120, 177
acute back pain: causes, 36-65
  coping with, 66-73
  exercises, 154, 156, 157-64
adaptive response training, 182
adhesions, ligaments, 47
adolescent osteochondritis, *56*, 57
ageing, 58-61, 99-100
alcohol, 49, 65, 76
Alexander technique, 127, 131-2, *132*, 133, 136
allergies, 109
  food, 49, 135
alternative therapies, 74-5, 127-35
anabolic steroids, 109
anaesthetics, local, 64, 103, 105, 107, 108
analgesics, 76, 101-2, 109
ankylosing spondylitis, 63, *63*, 77, 78, 93, 102
  exercises for, *164-6*
anti-depressants, 109, 181
anti-inflammatory drugs, 102, 109
antibiotics, 64
anxiety, 178, 181
arachnoiditis, 64, 79
arm pain, diagnosis, *34-5*
armchairs, getting out of, *73*
  see also sitting posture
aromatic oils, 72
arthritis, 64
  see also osteoarthritis; rheumatoid arthritis
arthrography, facet, 80
aspirin, 71, 72, 101, 109
autogenics, 180
autonomic nervous system, 94
autotraction, 87-8, *88*
avulsion, 52, *53*

B

babies, caring for, 149-51
back strengthening exercises, *169*
Back School, 75, 91
bacterial infections, 63
Balans chair, *141*
bathrooms, adapting, 147
baths, 70-1, 147
bed traction, 87
beds: boards, 68
  getting out of, *73*
  making, 148
  posture in, 142-4
  resting in, 68-70
bioenergetics, 127, 133-4
blood tests, 77, 78
bones: ageing, 58-9
  bone scans, 80-1
  diseases, 78
  infections, 63
  osteophytes, 59, *59*, 61, *62*
  osteoporosis, 58, *58*, 103
  Paget's disease, *58*, 59
braces, 90, *90*
brachialgia, 42-3, *42*, 59, 102, 107
brain, deep brain stimulators, 185
breathing exercises, 68, *166*
brucellosis, 64
bruising, coccyx, 53

C

cancer, 63, 93
cars, driving posture, 141-2
cartilage, vertebrae, 20
central canal stenosis, 61-2, *62*
  treatment for, 111, 112-13
cerebro-spinal fluid, *22*, 23
cervical collars, 89, *89*
cervical spondylosis, 116-17
cervical vertebrae, 18
chairs: getting out of, *73*
  posture in, 140-1, *140*, *141*
chemonucleolysis, 108-9
children, caring for, 149-51
chiropractic, 74-5, 92-3, 98-9, *99*
chronic back pain, causes, 36-65
chronic muscular tension, 49, 95
chymopapain, 64, 101, 108
clothes, 72, *73*, 147
coccydinia, 53, 116
coccyx, 17, 53, 116
codeine, 71, 101, 102, 109
coffee, 49, 177
collars, 88-9, *89*

compressed nerves, 41-3, *41*, *42*, 61-2
  see also sciatica *and* brachialgia
congenital defects, spinal, 57, 62, *62*
constipation, 76, 87, 94
continuous traction, 87
corsets, 61, 88-9, *89*, 90, 138
corticosteroids, 102, 103
cortisone, 43, 84, 102, 109
counter-irritants, 72
cricked neck *see* wry neck
crush fractures, 52-3, *53*, 58
cryocautery, 108
CT scans, 4 ,, 78, 81, *81*
cycling, 154

D

decompression surgery, 55, 59, 61, 62, 112-13, *113*
degenerative diseases, 77
  see also ageing
degenerative spondylolisthesis, 55
depression, 178, 181
diagnosis, 28, *29-35*, 36, 74-81, 82
diathermy, short wave, 85
disc prolapse *see* disc protrusion
disc protrusions, 37-41
  causes of, *38*
  central canal stenosis, 61
  chronic disc prolapse, 40-1
  epidural injections, 105-6
  exercises for, 156
  in the lower back, 38-9, *39*, 40
  manipulation, 94, 96
  in the mid back, 39, *39*
  in the neck, 39-41, *39*, 116
  sciatica and brachialgia, 42-3
  surgery, 64, 110-12, *112*
  types of, 37, *37*
discectomy, 110, 111-12, *112*
discitis, 64
discography, 80, *80*
discs: ageing, 58
  degeneration, 59, *60*
  herniated, 37, *37*
  infections, 64
  structure and function, 20-1, *20*, *21*
  traction, 85-8
  see also disc protrusions
  diseases, 63-4, 77
doctors, 74-8, *76*
draughts, cold, 49
driving, posture, 141-2
drug treatment, 71, 76, 101-3, 109, 177, 181
dural sheath, 23, 64

E

electrical stimulation, 183-5, *183*
electromyography, 79
electronic equipment, physiotherapy, 84-5
EMG feedback, 179-80
emotional reactions to pain, 178
encephalins, 122, 177, 183
endorphins, 122, 177, 183
epidural injections, 43, 105-7, *106*
epidural root fibrosis, 42, 43, *43*
epidural venography, 79-80
epidurography, 80
erythrocyte sedimentation rate, 77
exercise, 12-13, 154-70
  after acute attacks, 66, 72, 154
  for ankylosing spondylitis, *164-6*
  effects on discs, 21
  for the lower back, *157-62*
  for the neck, *163-4*
  sports, 152-3
  strengthening exercises, *166-70*

F

facet arthrography, 80
facet joints: acupuncture, 122
  disease, 60-1
  exercises, 156, *158*
  injections, 108
  spinal fusion, 113, *114*
  strain/malalignment, 44-5, *44*, 95
  structure, 19-20, *20*
  surgery, 111
  traction, 85-6
facetectomy, 59, *113*
Feldenkrais technique, 132, 133
fevers, 64, 65
fibrositis *see* trigger points
flu, 28, 65
food allergies, 49, 135
Fowler position, *69*, 70, 143
fracture dislocation, 117
fractures, vertebrae, 52-3, *53*, 55, *58*, 77, 110, 117
freeze injury techniques, 61, 108
functional scoliosis, 95-6
fusion operation, 47, 55, 61, 113-15, *114*

G

gall-bladder disorders, 65
gardening, 148, *149*
gate control theory, 176-7, *176*
gluteus maximus muscle, *24*
gynaecological disorders, 65
  relieving pain, 155

H

Harrington rod, 115, *115*
hamstrings, 13
  stretching exercises, *160-2*

headaches, 51, 98-9
heart attacks, 65
heat treatment, 70-1, 83-4
hollow back, 51
homeopathy, 127, 134-5
hormones: osteoporosis, 59
  pain-inhibiting, 122, 177, 183-5
housework, 146-8
hydrotherapy, 90-1
hypermobility, 51
hypnotherapy, 127-9, 177, 180

I

ice packs, 71
incontinence, 67
infections, 63, 64, 65, 77, 110, 111
inflammation, 63-4, 71, 77, 78
injections, 50, 51, 60, 103-8
injuries, spinal, 52-3
insomnia, 182
intercostal muscles, *24*
interferential therapy, 85
invalids, caring for, 151
inversion traction, 47, 55, 86-7, *86*
isometric exercises, 167, *170*

J

joints: ankylosing spondylitis, 63, *63*
  degenerative diseases, 77
  degenerative spondylolisthesis, 55
  facet joint disease, 60-1
  hypermobility, 51
  ligaments, 23, *23*
  manipulation, 94-5
  physiotherapy, 83
  strain and malalignment, 44-6, *44*, *46*
  structure and function, 19-20, *20*
  traction, 85-6
  see also facet joints

K

kidney disorders, 65
kissing spines, 51
kitchens, adapting, 146, *147*

L

laminectomy, 110, *113*
lateral canal stenosis, 42, 59, *59*
  surgery for, 111, 112-13
lateral decompression, 59, 61, 112-3, *113*
leg exercises, 23, 156, *160-2*, *168-9*
leg pain: diagnosis, 29-31
  exercises, 156
lifting techniques, *145*, 146
ligaments, 23, *23*
  ageing, 58
  ankylosing spondylitis, 63, *63*
  injections, 103, 104-5, *105*
  injuries, 47-8, *48*

postural pain, 50-1
sclerosant therapy, 46, 47, 55, 59, 60, 61, 104-5, *104*
  slack or strained, 47
lower back: acupressure, *174*
  diagnosis of pain, *29-31*
  disc protrusions, 38-9, *39*, 40
  exercises, 156, *157-62*
  facet joint disease, 60
  instability, 113, 156
  joint strain and malalignment, 44-5
  ligament injuries, 47
  manipulation, 94
  stress fractures, 52
  vertebrae, 18, *19*, 57
lumbago, 36, 38
  acupressure, *174*
  acupuncture, 120, *123*
  drug treatment, 102
  exercises, *158*
  manipulation, 94, 96, 97
lumbar puncture, 79
lumbar spine *see* lower back
lung infections, 65
lying hamstring stretch, *161*
lying positions, 68-70, *69*, 142-4, *143*

M

Maitlands method, physiotherapy, 82, 83, *83*
malaligned joints, 44-6, *44*
manipulation, 39, 40, 42, 44, 45, 46, 48, 60, 82, 84, 92-100, *97-100*
massage: acupressure, 125-6, *174*
  giving a massage, 172, *173*
  pain relief, 71
  physiotherapy, 82, 83, 84
  relaxation, 50, 172, *173*
mattresses, 68, 143
medicines, 71, 76, 101-3, 109
meditation, 127, 129-30, 180
Melzack, Prof. Ronald, 120, 176
meninges, 21
menopause, 58
menstruation, 65
  relieving pain, 155
mentholatum, 72
meridians, acupuncture, 118-19, *119*
microfractures, 52, *53*
microsurgery, 111-12
mid back: diagnosis of pain, *32-3*
  disc protrusions, 39, *39*
  facet joint disease, 61
  joint strain and malalignment, 45
migraine, 94, 98-9
Milwaukee brace, *90*
mobilizing exercises, *159-60*
morphine, 101, 109, 177
moving without pain, 72, *73*
moxibustion, 125, *125*
muscles: chronic tension, 95
  deterioration, 67
  exercises, 154-70
  injections, 103

massage, 172, *173*
muscle relaxants, 102, 109
physiotherapy, 83
postural pain, 50-1
relaxation, 68, 70-2, 171, 179-81
sports, 152-3
strains, 48-50
structure, 23-6, *24, 25*
tension, 49-50
myelography, 43, 64, 78-9, *79*
myofascial dysfunction *see* trigger
points

N

narcotics, 101-2, 109, 184
neck: collars, 88-9
diagnosis of pain, *34-5*
disc protrusions, 38, *39*, 40-1
drug treatment, 102
exercises, 156, *163-5, 170*
facet joint disease, 61
joint strain and malalignment, 45
ligament injuries, 47
lying posture, 143, *144*
manipulation, 94-5
muscular tension, 49
pillows, 143, *144*
postural pain, 51
resting positions, 68, *69*, 70
surgery, 116-17
traction, 86, 87, 94-5
trigger points, 49-50, *50*
whiplash injuries, 47-8, *48*
wry neck, 40, 45, 94, 156
Neck Schools, 91
nerves: central canal stenosis, 61-2, *62*
compressed, 41-3, *41*, *42*, 61-2
decompression surgery, 112-13
disc protrusions, 67
electrical stimulation, 183-5, *183*
gate control theory, 176-7, *176*
manipulation, 94
muscle stimulation, 26
nerve block injection, 107-8, *107*
nerve root pain, 41
spinal cord, 21-3, *22*
spinal injuries, 52
stenosis of the spinal canal, 59, *59*
transcutaneous nerve stimulation,
85, 183-4, *183*
neuro-stimulation, 183-5, *183*
numbness, 67

O

oils, aromatic, 72
osteoarthritis, 58, 80
treatment for, 94, 108, 122
osteochondritis, adolescent, *56*, 57
osteopathy, 74-5, 92-3, 96, 97
osteophytes, 58, 59, *59*, 61, *62*, 77
surgery for, 112
osteoporosis, 52, 58, *58*, 103
see also crush fractures

P

Paget's disease, *58*, 59
pain: coping with, 179-85
describing, 75
pain clinics, 75, 182
pain gate, 122, *176*
pain-killers, 76, 101-2, 109
pain relief, 70-2
perception of, 175-9
pancreas, inflammation, 65
panic attacks, 181
paracetamol, 71, 101, 109
pelvic block, 152
pelvis, 27, *46*
posture, 138-9, *138*
pethidine, 101, 109
phobias, 181
physiotherapy, 48, 50, 59, 60-1, 75,
82-91
pillows, 68, *69*, *144*
pins and needles, 40, 41, 42, 67
pleurisy, 65
pneumonia, 65
poliomyelitis, 26
posture, 12, 136-44
Alexander technique, 131-2, *132*,
136
bioenergetics, 133-4
driving posture, 141-2
and emotional moods, 16
lying down, *69*, 142-4, *143*
muscular tension, 49
postural pain, 50-1
sitting posture, 139-41
standing posture, 138-9
pre-menstrual tension, 94
pregnancy, 45, 47, 137, 138, 150
relieving back pain, 155
pressure on the spine, *141*
prolotherapy, 104
psoas muscles, *25*, 139
psychological factors, 14-16, 49, 175
psychotherapy, 133-4

R

radiculography, 78
relaxation, 67-70, 171-2, *173*, 179-81
rest, 67-70, *71*
rheumatoid arthritis, 63, 64, 77
treatment for, 102, 134, 135
rhizolysis, 108
rib lesions, 95
risk factors, 10-16
rubs, 72

S

sacroiliac joint, 45-6, *46*, 63, 77, 95
sacrum, 17
Scheuermann's disease, *56*, 57
sciatic scoliosis, 55
sciatica, 36
acupressure, *174*

acupuncture, 120, 122
causes, 41-2, *42*, 59
chronic sciatica, 42-3
drug treatment, 102
epidural injections, 105
exercises, *157*
manipulation, 95
nerve blocks, 107
surgery, 110-11
traction, 87
sclerosant injections, 46, 47, 55, 59,
60, 61, 104-5, *104*
scoliosis, 12, 55-7, *56*
treatment for, *90*, 95-6, 115-16,
115
self-hypnosis, 128, 129, 180
sexual activity, 151-2
shiatsu, 125-6, *174*
short wave diathermy, 85
shoulder pain, diagnosis, *34-5*
sitting posture, 70, 139-41, *139-41*
sleep problems, 182
slipped disc *see* disc protrusions
specialists, 77-81
spina bifida occulta, 57
spinal cord: stenosis, 59, *59*, 61-2,
62, 111, 112-13
structure and function, 17, 21-3,
22
violent injuries, 52
spinal fusion, 47, 55, 61, 113-15, *114*
spine: congenital defects, 57
structural defects, 55-7, *56*
structure and function, 17-27,
18-25
violent injuries, 52-3
see also vertebrae
spinous processes: fractures, 52
kissing spines, 51
structure, 19, *19*
spondylolisthesis, 54-5, *54*, 77
treatment for, 104, 111, 112-14
spondylolysis, 54, *54*, 77
spondylosis, 58
sports, 12, 152-3
standing posture, 137-9, *137*
stenosis of the spinal canal, 59, *59*,
61-2, *62*, 111, 112-13
steroids, 43, 64, 102, 103, 105, 109
stomach ulcers, 65, 71
strains: joints, 44-6, *44*, *46*
ligaments, 47
muscles, 48-50, 156
strengthening exercises, *166-70*
stress, 16, 49
stress fractures, 52
stress inoculation therapy, 182-3
stretching exercises, 50, *160-2*, *164*
structural defects, 55
subluxation *see* malaligned joints
surgery, 110-17, *112-15*
arachnoiditis, 64
central canal stenosis, 62
coccydinia, 53, 116
decompression, 112-3, *112*

disc protrusions, 39, 43, 110-12, *112*
discectomy, 110-12, *112*
facet joint disease, 61
failure of, 117
ligament injuries, 47
neck, 61, 116-17
osteophytes, 59
scoliosis, 115-16, *115*
spinal fusion, 57, 113-15, *114*
spondylolisthesis, 55
stenosis, 112-13, *113*
sway back syndrome, 51
swimming, 91, 154
synovial fluid, 20

T

tail-bone *see* coccyx
tension, muscular, 49-50
tension headaches, 51
thoracic vertebrae, 18, *19*
tomograms, 78, 81, *81*
torticollis, *see* wry neck
traction, 39, 40, 42, 47, 55, 60, 61, 85-8
  autotraction, 87-8, *88*
  inversion traction, 86, *86*
tranquillizers, 181

transcutaneous nerve stimulation (TNS), 85, 183-4, *183*
trapezius muscle, *24*
tricyclics, 181
trigger points, *50*
  acupuncture, 121, 122
  causes, 45, 49-50
  exercises, 156
  injections, 103
  ultrasound treatment, 84
tuberculosis, 64
tumours, 63, 77, 110, 111
twisting exercises, *160, 165*

U

ulcers, stomach, 65, 71
ultrasound: physiotherapy, 50, 84
  scans, 81
uterus, prolapse, 65

V

valium, 177, 181
vertebrae: adolescent osteochondritis, *56*, 57
central canal stenosis, 61-2, *62*
fracture dislocation, 117
fractures, 52-3, *53*, 55

joint strain and malalignment, 44-5
osteophytes, 58, 59, 112
spondylolisthesis, 54-5, *54*
spondylolysis, 54, *54*
structure and function, 17-21, *18*, *19*
vertebral artery, 89
vertebro-basilar syndrome, 89
vibrators, 71-2
virus infections, 65

W

wedge compressions, 53, *53*, 95
whiplash injuries, 47-8, *48*, 89, 95, 98-9, *98, 99*
womb, prolapse, 65
women: gynaecological disorders, 65
  menopause, 58
  menstruation, 65, 155
  osteoporosis, 58
  pregnancy, 45, 47, 138, 155
work, and back pain, 13-14, 177-8
wry neck, 40, 45, 94, 156

X

X-rays, 36, 52, 53, 77-81, *79-81*, 82

ACKNOWLEDGMENTS

Author's acknowledgments
First and foremost I am indebted to the late Dr James Cyriax, founder of the system of orthopaedic medicine, who has inspired countless doctors and physiotherapists over the world by his tireless and lifelong dedication to the diagnosis and treatment of the aches and pain that afflict so many people. Without his contribution to my career, I would probably not be on the starting block nor would this book be possible.

Thanks are due in particular to Dr James Hawkins MB, BChir (Cantab), Trustee for the British Holistic Medical Association, for his help and research of the material for the section on acupuncture and hypnosis. I am grateful to: Tina Everett MCSP for her contributions to the chapter on physiotherapy and self-help for women, pregnancy, and the relaxation procedure; Vivienne Lyle DO, DAc, DC, for her contributions on chiropractic and acupuncture; and Tom Falkner ND, DO, for his help with osteopathic methods and treatment. In addition I would like to thank my two secretaries, Pat Brittin and Lesley Howe for their hard work, support and their patience with a demanding author. Acknowledgments must also go to Gill Needham, librarian at Milton Keynes Hospital for digging out reference material, and to the Back Pain Association and The Royal National Orthopaedic Hospital X-Ray Library for supplying photographs. Last but not least I must thank all those thousands of patients who, through their suffering, have helped to provide me with experience, understanding and encouragement to proceed.

Dorling Kindersley would like to thank: Diana Mansour for her editorial help; Fred and Kathy Gill for proof-reading; Hilary Bird for the index; Tim Hammond for modelling the exercises; Georgie Duff and Jasper Humphreys for demonstrating the Maitlands Mobilization technique; and Iona McGlashan for design assistance.

Illustrators
John Woodcock, Nick Hall, Line and Line
Photographer
Paul Fletcher
X-ray sources
□ pp. 54, 56, 58, 79, 80, 81 reproduced by courtesy of the Institute of Orthopaedics, London
□ p. 56 scoliosis: Milton Keynes General Hospital
Typesetting
Rowland Phototypesetting (London) Ltd
Airedale Graphics
Reproduction
Reprocolour Llovet Barcelona SA